Introduction to
U.S. Health Policy

Related Benjamin Cummings Health Titles

Anspaugh/Ezell, *Teaching Today's Health*, Sixth Edition (2001)

Buckingham, *A Primer on International Health* (2001)

Cottrell/Girvan/McKenzie, *Principles & Foundations of Health Promotion and Education*, Second Edition (2002)

Donatelle, *Access to Health*, Seventh Edition (2002)

Donatelle, *Health: The Basics*, Fourth Edition (2001)

Donnelly, Elburne, Kittleson, *Mental Health: Dimensions of Self-Esteem and Emotional Well-Being* (2001)

Girdano/Dusek/Everly, *Controlling Stress and Tension*, Sixth Edition (2001)

Karren/Hafen/Smith/Frandsen, *Mind/Body Health*, Second Edition (2002)

McKenzie/Smeltzer, *Planning, Implementing, and Evaluating Health Promotion Programs: A Primer*, Third Edition (2001)

Neutens/Rubinson, *Research Techniques for the Health Sciences*, Third Edition (2002)

Reagan/Brookins-Fisher, *Community Health in the 21st Century*, Second Edition (2002)

Seaward, *Health of the Human Spirit: Spiritual Dimensions for Personal Health* (2001)

Skinner, *Promoting Health through Organizational Change* (2002)

Please visit us at **www.aw.com/bc** for more information about these and other Benjamin Cummings Health titles.

Introduction to
U.S. Health Policy

The Organization, Financing, and Delivery of Health Care in America

Donald A. Barr, MD, PhD

Stanford University

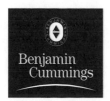

San Francisco   Boston   New York
Cape Town   Hong Kong   London   Madrid   Mexico City
Montreal   Munich   Paris   Singapore   Sidney   Tokyo   Toronto

Publisher: Daryl Fox
Acquisitions Editor: Deirdre McGill
Publishing Assistant: Michelle Cadden
Managing Editor: Wendy Earl
Production Editor: Janet Vail
Copy Editor: Anita Wagner
Proofreader: Anne Friedman
Cover and Text Designer: Brad Greene
Cover Photographer: David Bradford
Manufacturing Buyers: Megan Cochran, Stacey Weinberger
Marketing Manager: Sandra Lindelof

Library of Congress Cataloging-in-Publication Data
Barr, Donald A.
     Introduction to U.S. Health Policy: the organization, financing, and delivery
of health care in America / Donald A. Barr.
          p. cm.
     Includes bibliographical references and index
     ISBN 0-205-32419-3
     1. Medical policy--United States. 2. Health policy--United States. 3. Health
planning--United States. 4. Medicine--United States. I. Title: Introduction to US
health policy. II. Title

     RA393.B335 2002
     362.l'0973--dc21

                                                                2001043693

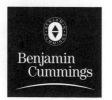

ISBN 0-205-32419-3

1 2 3 4 5 6 7 8 9 10–DVA–05 04 03 02 01

www.aw.com/bc

FOR DEBRA

About the Author

Donald Barr received his M.D. from the University of California, San Francisco and his Ph.D. in sociology from Stanford University. He is an associate professor of sociology and human biology at Stanford and is the founder and director of Stanford's undergraduate health policy curriculum. His research focuses on the effect of the organizational structure of the medical care delivery system on the quality of primary care.

Dr. Barr brings to this book the unique perspective of being both a practicing physician and an academic sociologist. He has experienced first-hand the sweeping changes that have occurred in the organizing and financing of health care through 25 years of medical practice in Northern California. As an experienced researcher and writer in the area of health policy, he is able to combine a broad understanding of the social and economic forces affecting health care with an appreciation of the effects of these changes on the quality of care experienced by patients and practitioners alike.

Dr. Barr is a member of the American Public Health Association, the Academy for Health Services Research and Health Policy, and the American Sociological Association.

Contents

Foreword

Introduction to U.S. Health Policy

By Philip R. Lee, M.D.

Health care in the United States is a matter of growing concern, not just to the health professionals who provide the care but to employers who purchase care, public officials at all levels of government, union members who bargain for benefits, the millions without health insurance, and the broader public. In this thorough and engaging book, Dr. Donald Barr has brought this complex yet critically important topic to a new generation of readers.

In this textbook on the organization, financing, and delivery of health care in America, Dr. Barr brings the perspective of a clinician with 30 years of experience and a social scientist (his doctorate is in sociology) who has studied the health care system for more than a decade. This book is built on his highly successful teaching record in the Program in Human Biology at Stanford University, where Dr. Barr has brought the subject of health care in America, previously a topic thought to be the province of professionals and graduate academics, to hundreds of undergraduates.

This book is a practical, in-depth guide to the factors that have shaped health care in America, as well as the consequences of our uniquely American approach to health care. He explores the roles of medicine and nursing as shapers of the system as well as providers of care. He examines the peculiar American obsession with medical care as a market good rather than a public good, the problems that have resulted from the rise of managed care (particularly for-profit plans), the impact of this system on those without health insurance, and the multiple factors in addition to insurance that affect access to care.

This is a wonderful introduction to health care in America. It should be a valuable resource for undergraduate students, for health professionals and graduate students, and for those who just want to be informed by a stimulating and fresh look at health care in America.

Preface

This book is about the United States health care system. It provides an introduction to the various organizations and institutions that make our system work (or not work, as the case may be). It identifies historical forces that have brought us to our current state of health care and examines the way in which the need of the American people for health care services is sometimes met and sometimes not.

Over the last decade especially there has been a growing debate over the quality and adequacy of health care in America. "This country has the best health care system in the world" is a claim often heard in the political discourse over health care. "This country has one of the worst health care systems among industrialized nations" is a frequent complaint raised in opposition to the current system.

The irony of U.S. health care, and a principal message of this book, is that both claims are simultaneously true. From one perspective we have the best health care available anywhere. From another, equally valid perspective we are close to worst among developed countries in the way we structure our health care system. Which perspective one adopts depends on the measure of quality one chooses.

This seeming paradox is illustrated by the way health care is provided in the communities adjoining the office in which this book is being written. Approximately 500 yards to the north is Stanford University Medical Center, a world leader in technological sophistication in medical care. Doctors there, who are among the best in the world, are able to perform remarkable feats, such as lifesaving organ transplants or reattachment of severed hands. The physician-scientists at the Packard Children's Hospital are able to save amazingly tiny, premature babies weighing less than this book. Specialist physicians in the emergency room are able to reverse heart attacks and strokes after they have already happened. Nowhere in the world is a higher level of advanced medical care available.

Approximately 2 miles to the east of this office is the community of East Palo Alto. The population of East Palo Alto is predominantly low-income, predominantly nonwhite, and to a large extent without health insurance. Many of the people there have no regular source of medical care. When they or their children become ill, the only source of care available is often the emergency room at Stanford Hospital, where doctors in training will see and treat them in between treating patients with heart attacks or major traumatic injuries. If patients from East Palo Alto need to be hospitalized, those with no insurance and no means for paying for care out of pocket are not allowed treatment in Stanford Hospital. Rather, they are referred to a county hospital, several miles away. East Palo Alto has a high rate of premature babies; violence is a major health problem; diseases such as diabetes or high blood pressure often go untreated; some children go without needed checkups and immunizations.

This is the dilemma of health care in America.

As this book describes, we spend more on health care, both overall and per capita, than any other country in the world. Yet the health of our society, measured by indices such as infant mortality and life expectancy, and our access to care is worse than nearly all other industrialized countries.

Two broad forces contribute to the relatively poor state of health in the United States: socioeconomic factors such as education, poverty, and lifestyle, and the quality of our health care system. It may in fact be that socioeconomic factors have more to do with the overall health of our society than does our system of health care. This book, though, looks only at the latter—at our health care system.

It has been health care, not health, that has focused national attention and stirred national discourse for the past several years. During the debate over the Clinton health reform proposals in 1993–1994 we had a graphic illustration of how our health care system is made up of various organizations and groups that often can't agree on how the system should be structured. This was not the first time we tried to initiate broad reform of the health care system in this country. In the 1930s a national health care plan was proposed as part of Social Security. It was seen as too far-reaching, and was dropped from the plan to ensure passage. In the years following World War II, President Truman proposed a national system of health insurance, but was defeated by the forces of organized medicine. In the 1960s Congress adopted major policy reforms in the way we finance health care for the elderly and the poor, but stopped short of comprehensive national reform. In the 1970s, facing for the first time the rapidly rising cost of health care that characterized the last part of the twentieth century, Congress came close to adopting comprehensive national reform, only to back away in the wake of the Watergate scandal.

As health care costs appear again to be rising, and more and more people are left without health insurance, the beginning of the twenty-first century will see the same problems that confronted the end of the twentieth century. Congress no doubt will try again to deal with the growing problem of health care. Unless something on the horizon changes, they will probably pass only incremental changes, as they have tended to do in the past. In all likelihood the problems of high cost, unequal access, and maintaining the quality of health care in America will remain. Whether as a health care professional who participates in the system, as an academician who studies the system, or as a patient who turns to the system for care, you, the reader of this book, will confront the questions swirling about health care again and again.

The debate over national health care reform often sidesteps the issue of balancing costs and benefits. As a consequence of expecting the most advanced, technological care, even when the added benefit of that care is modest relative to its cost, we have both increased the cost of care and excluded millions from access to care. How much can we as a country afford to spend on health care? Can we constrain the growth of health care expenditures and also improve access to care?

Who will find the answers or make the difficult choices? Physicians, health care administrators, and those responsible for the public sector will all play an important role in this process. However, many doctors and other health care professionals don't get adequate training in the knowledge and skills necessary to make informed choices about health care delivery.

In 1995, Drs. Ira Nash and Richard Pasternak reported their experience in interviewing applicants for one of the most competitive and prestigious fellowship training programs in the country. They found that nearly all the applicants had consistently high clinical qualifications. They then asked these young physicians, the future leaders of the medical profession, what they thought about the issue of health care reform.

> *We were shocked when we barely got a response. A few residents offered some brief insight into the scope of the challenge to reform. Fewer enunciated some broad goal of reform such as universal insurance coverage. None had any well-formed ideas about how to actually address these challenges or realize these goals, or could even render a reasoned opinion about somebody else's well-formed idea. . . . How can it be that the apparent "best and brightest" of*

internal medicine are on the intellectual sidelines of the debate over health sys-
tem reform?

     . . . If, as is now the case, we find time in medical school and residency
training to teach things that most physicians will never need to know, we
should find the teachers and the time to teach what nearly every physician will
soon need to know to help address the health care needs of the nation. (Nash,
IS and Pasternak, RC. *Physician, Educate Thyself. JAMA* 1995; 273(19):
1533–34.)

Medical science has been expanding steadily since the beginning of the
twentieth century. Initially, doctors had a fairly small core of knowledge
they needed to acquire. As scientists learned about bacteria and other
microorganisms, doctors needed to expand their base of knowledge to
include microbiology. When X-ray technology began to expand, doctors
needed also to learn the basics of radiology. In the 1960s and 1970s, as a
phenomenal number of new drugs were discovered, doctors needed to
learn more about pharmacology. Every time a new development has
occurred in medical practice, doctors have needed to expand their base of
knowledge to include the new area.

Another new area is developing, with at least as much significance for
the practice of medicine as others that came before it. This development is
the tremendous change we are seeing in the financing and organization of
health care and the profound consequences this change is having on health
care delivery. Just as doctors expanded the knowledge required for the
practice of medicine in the face of technological advances, many now suggest that health care professionals of all types need to expand their knowledge to include a familiarity with the health care delivery system and the
effects of alternative delivery methods on the outcomes of care. Whether
acquired as part of an undergraduate education or as part of the curriculum
of health profession schools, knowledge of health policy will be an important part of professional knowledge in the twenty-first century.

The purpose of this book is to provide the reader with just such knowledge. Developed from a course I have taught at Stanford University for several years, the book describes the historical, social, political, and economic
forces that have shaped our health care system and created the policy
dilemmas we face. The information offered in this book has proved to be of
interest to undergraduates, medical students, and practicing professionals
alike, all of which have participated in the course.

The book stops short of offering specific policy solutions to the many problems identified. Identifying and adopting policies to address these problems necessarily involves extended discussion and debate and a balancing of conflicting interests. Fortunately the reader has available a number of health policy journals that provide a forum for the analysis of potential policy solutions. I encourage the reader to supplement the material in this book by becoming familiar with journals such as *Health Affairs* (www.healthaffairs.org), *Milbank Quarterly* (www.milbank.org/quarterly.html), and the *Journal of Health Care Politics, Policy, and Law* (www.jhppl.org). An examination of current health reform options can easily be added to courses using this book, either through supplemental discussion sections or, in the format I have adopted, as a follow-up seminar.

Other resources

What Is Health Policy?

This book provides an introduction to health policy in the United States. The growing problems that have surrounded health care over the past several decades have created the field of health policy. Thirty years ago, few if any universities or professional schools had teaching or research programs in health policy. Today nearly every major university includes active programs in health policy. Academic journals specializing in health policy are increasingly numerous and well respected. The advent of the Internet has made an extensive library of health policy data and information immediately available to all with basic computer access.

As with any new academic discipline, there is not universal agreement as to what precisely constitutes the field of health policy. Overlapping interests among those in fields such as public health, health economics, and health services research have made agreement on a precise definition of health policy difficult to attain. This book hopes to address this problem by approaching health policy as the study of the way health care is organized, financed, and delivered. It does this by drawing on theories from fields such as economics, sociology, and organizational behavior to offer a view of the broad social forces that coalesce to create the structure of our system of health care and the problems inherent in it.

In its broadest sense health policy includes all those factors and forces that affect the health of the public. This book, however, focuses its study of health policy more on the structure of health care than on the health of a community or society.

allocation of resources is best left to the market mechanism + any interference reduces the efficiency of the economy

Flip side is capable markets are up of collective taking care such as worder

Health policy overlaps with health economics, but broadens its scope to include social and political processes affecting health care. Health policy and health services research have much in common; however, the latter tends to look more at specific clinical issues, such as the optimal way to treat coronary artery disease, while health policy looks at questions such as the optimal way to structure care overall.

Who Makes Health Policy?

The organizing, financing, and delivery of health care in America is affected by a broad range of forces, public as well as private, national as well as local. Congress and the federal health agencies within the executive branch have major roles in developing health policy. Federal laws such as Medicare and Medicaid that affect the financing of care have also reshaped health care organization and delivery in a number of ways. Rules established by the U.S. Department of Health and Human Services govern much of the health care that is provided in this country. The congressional system of committees and subcommittees plays a continuous role in monitoring the delivery of health care throughout the country and initiating reform when necessary.

States also play a major role in the organization and financing of health care. Most laws governing professional licensure and medical practice come from the states. Financing care for the poor has become largely the responsibility of the states.

Health policy, however, includes more than just the creation of governmental policies pertaining to health care. As discussed later in this book, private businesses play a major role, both as purchasers of health insurance and providers of health insurance, in driving recent changes in the way health care is organized, financed, and delivered. The shift to a market-based system of managed care was largely the result of the need to control costs. The effect this shift has had on the actual delivery of care at every level is profound.

The providers of care also play a large role in developing health policy. The American Medical Association (AMA), the private organization representing physicians, has been one of the most powerful forces behind the creation of the private practice, fee-for-service model of health care delivery that came to dominate the health care system for much of the twentieth century. Other providers, competing with the AMA, formed cooperative associations of doctors and hospitals as an alternative to fee-for-service care.

These alternative, prepaid systems created the model on which the concept of the health maintenance organization (HMO) was based.

Local communities also play a role in creating health policy. Community hospitals, community clinics, and local government health departments continue to play a major role in the organization and delivery of care at the local level.

So the creation of health policy is more than simply passing laws. It is the coalescence of forces on multiple levels, representing multiple interests and constituencies, to organize and finance a system to deliver health care to the American people.

Structure of the Book

The 12 chapters of the book present the dilemma of American health care, describe its basic structure, and identify recent changes and trends in the system. For each chapter a series of "Key Concepts" summarizes the way social, economic, and political factors have acted to shape health care delivery in this country, either historically or concurrently. By fully understanding these concepts the reader will have developed a comprehensive grasp of our system of care.

Chapter 1 starts with a brief historical background about some of the important policy decisions our country has made over time that have created the system we now have. It provides data about the rising cost of health care in this country, and the burdens these costs place on both government and the private sector. It compares our country to other developed countries, both in the amount we spend on health care and the overall health of our societies.

Chapter 2 describes how the institutional norms and expectations that are unique to the United States have created a health care system that is also unique. As a means of comparison, it traces the history of the Canadian health care system and examines how fundamental cultural differences between U.S. and Canadian society are reflected in our health care systems.

Chapter 3 looks at the professional structure of American health care. It describes the history of the medical profession, examining such issues as the number of physicians in practice and their practice specialty. It covers the history of the nursing profession and the evolving role of advanced practice nurses. Finally, it examines the structure of hospitals and other types of specialized referral centers.

Chapter 4 addresses the various ways health insurance can be structured. It provides a close look at the health maintenance organization, or HMO. It looks at the evolution of the Kaiser-Permanente system, for years the nation's largest HMO. It then describes the emergence over the last several years of newer types of HMOs and various other types of managed care organizations.

Chapters 5 and 6 explore the two principal government health care programs: Medicare and Medicaid. Established in the 1960s, these programs simultaneously extended health insurance coverage to millions of Americans who were previously without insurance coverage, and set off the escalation in health care costs that continue to plague us today. It describes some of the policy questions confronting Medicare, and recent efforts by several states to restructure their Medicaid system to both constrain costs and broaden coverage.

Chapter 7 moves on to a discussion of the managed care revolution and the widespread introduction of the for-profit motive into health care delivery. It distinguishes between the concepts of managed care and managed competition. It asks how the rapid shift to for-profit based managed care will affect health care delivery.

Chapter 8 covers changes that have taken place in the Medicare system in response to the widening availability of HMOs. It describes some of the weaknesses and problems that have been identified with the system of Medicare HMOs, and recent steps Congress has taken to reform this program.

Chapter 9 explores the often hidden side of American health care: our system of long-term health care. It covers a variety of long-term care options, including nursing homes and home health care. It documents the expected surge in frail, elderly Americans who will soon be in need of long-term care services, and looks at alternative ways of providing and financing long-term care.

Chapter 10 brings up the issue of the uninsured: the 44 million Americans who are without any type of health insurance coverage and as a result lack access to many types of basic medical care. It finds that a large majority of the uninsured are not people who are poor and unemployed, but rather are people in families with at least one adult who works on a regular basis. It looks at the success and problems of two different efforts to reduce the number of uninsured: Hawaii's employer mandate for the provision of health insurance to workers, and the State Children's Health

Insurance Program enacted by the federal government to reduce the number of children without health insurance.

Chapter 11 looks at social factors other than health insurance that affect health care delivery and the access to health care. It asks, what are some of the other factors that impede people's access to health care even after financial constraints have been removed? It describes how forces such as culture, ethnicity, and social class can independently affect access to care.

Chapter 12 puts the lessons learned in the previous 11 chapters into a single, unified model of our current health care dilemma. It suggests that forces of cost, quality, and access compete for preeminence in the health policy arena, and that the recent interjection of the for-profit motive has complicated the model and made a solution more difficult. It proposes an ethical heuristic that physicians and other health professionals can use to navigate the currents of for-profit health care. It explores the issue of health care rationing and the lessons that can be learned from the Oregon Health Plan for Medicaid, the country's first attempt at the explicit rationing of health care services as a means to expand access.

It is my hope that at the completion of this book, the reader will gain an appreciation of how health care in America in all its complexity represents a fundamental dilemma: How much health care can we afford and who will have access to that care? I will consider the book a success if, as result of this appreciation, the reader will be in a better position to contribute to solving that dilemma.

Donald A. Barr, M.D., Ph.D.

Acknowledgments

There are many people without whose input, support, and guidance this book would never have been a reality. I gratefully acknowledge what they have given me.

Adam, Isaac, and Deagon continue to amaze me in many ways and make my life complete.

Russ Fernald and Bill Durham, directors of the Program in Human Biology at Stanford, gave me the opportunity to develop the ideas contained in the book.

Dick Scott and John Meyer helped me realize how important institutions are in a variety of settings, especially health care.

Victor Fuchs showed me how to use economic principles in complex social situations.

Jim March made it clear that quixotic isn't necessarily a bad thing to be.

Phil Lee introduced me to the field of health policy more than 30 years ago and continues to help me improve my understanding of this crucially important field of study.

CHAPTER 1

Health, Health Care, and the Market Economy

Key Concepts

- Two policies established early in the twentieth century had major effects on our system of care and contributed to our current problems:

  Approaching medical care as a market commodity

  Granting sovereignty to the medical profession over the organization and financing of medical care

- If the rising cost of health care as a percentage of GDP is not slowed, the impacts on our economy will be substantial:

  Investment in other sectors of the economy will shrink.

  American businesses will be at a competitive disadvantage with foreign competitors.

  Federal, state, and local governments will have to either raise taxes or go increasingly in debt.

- The United States spends more on health care than any other country in the world. Despite this high level of expenditure, we have one of the lowest levels of overall health of any developed country. The only measure of health in which our country excels is the additional number of years an 80-year-old person can expect to live.

- Among developed countries, there is little correlation between the amount a country spends on health care and the overall level of health of that country. The health of a society has more to do with the level of education and income than it does with health care.

1

The Unique History of Health Care in America

As a people we are accustomed to hospital service; we look upon that service no longer as a luxury which we may buy, but rather as an inherent right. The humblest patient is entitled to the best of medical service. In the last twenty years especially this idea has taken hold of us. We regard the right to health today much as we regard the right to life. (John G. Bowman, Director, Board of Regents, American College of Surgeons)

This statement, made by the director of one of the most prestigious groups of physicians in the United States, bespeaks a commitment on the part of the medical profession and the country to approach health care as a basic right for all individuals. As part of the health care debate that has been taking place over the last several years in this country, many people have advocated this position as the basis for future reform. Dr. Bowman, however, made this statement in 1918. As more than 40 million uninsured Americans who are without access to health care will attest, his vision served as a poor predictor of the path health care in this country would follow. The history of American health care in the twentieth century is more accurately reflected by the following statement, published in a major medical journal in 1971.

Medical care is neither a right nor a privilege: it is a service that is provided by doctors and others to people who wish to purchase it. (Sade 1971, p. 1289)

Viewing medical care as a market commodity that can be bought or sold, rather than a social good that should be made available to all people, is a uniquely American policy position. In the words of economist Uwe Reinhardt,

Americans have . . . decided to treat health care as essentially a private consumer good of which the poor might be guaranteed a basic package, but which is otherwise to be distributed more and more on the basis of ability to pay. (Reinhardt and Relman 1986, p. 23)

We are alone among industrialized nations in approaching health care in this market-oriented way. All other developed countries have adopted national health plans that ensure access to basic medical care for their citizens. These plans range from fully socialized systems such as that in Great Britain to systems such as Canada's, in which all doctors are in private medical practice.[1]

---

[1] A short time ago, there was a second developed country that approached medical care as a market commodity. In that country, those citizens without the ability to pay for it had little if any access to care. As a result of a major restructuring of the country's government, it adopted the policy of health care for all as a basic right, leaving the United States alone in treating it as a market good. This other country was South Africa.

A second national policy decision has had equally profound effects on the way health care evolved in the United States. This was the decision made in the early part of the twentieth century to vest in the medical profession substantial authority over the organization and financing as well as the practice of medical care. At the beginning of the twentieth century the American medical profession was a complex array of practitioners from a variety of educational backgrounds with a variety of knowledge and skills. There were no standards, either legal or ethical, that maintained a consistent level of quality in the way physicians practiced medicine.

In response to what was perceived as a national crisis, a prestigious commission was appointed to make recommendations about a thorough restructuring of medical education. In 1910 the commission published its recommendations in its report, *Medical Education in the United States and Canada*, often referred to as the Flexner report. Based on the views expounded in this report, state and local governments increasingly relied on the American Medical Association (AMA) (the principal professional association of physicians) and on the AMA's affiliated state and local medical associations to guide the restructuring of medical practice. (For a more comprehensive discussion of this period in the history of American medicine, see Paul Starr's Pulitzer Prize-winning book, *The Social Transformation of American Medicine*.)

The rise in the sovereignty of the American medical profession was based on a somewhat idealized view of physicians. Consistent with the increasing legitimacy of science and technology common during that time, physicians were typically seen as altruistic agents who possessed valuable scientific knowledge and technical skills (Parsons 1951, 1975). Their role as social agents was guided by a code of medical ethics that placed the utmost importance on acting at all times in the best interest of the patient. They could be trusted to make decisions on behalf of the patient in a paternalistic manner, acting always as a disinterested agent on the patient's behalf. It was this view of the medical profession that led state and local governments to vest in physicians and their professional organizations considerable authority over medical education and the practice of medicine.

Although this view of physicians as agents of reason exerted substantial influence over governmental policy toward medical care, a historical examination of the ways in which physicians' professional organizations have actually exerted the authority given to them offers a very different picture (Freidson 1970). Physicians were granted this authority because of their specialized knowledge and skills, but they often used this power to further their own ends. In this view of physicians as agents of power, the medical profession is seen as using its control over knowledge to limit entry into the profession and to maintain political sovereignty over the system of

Table 1.1   Two Ways to Look at the Medical Profession in the United States

Physicians as Agents of Reason[a]	Physicians as Agents of Power[b]
Authority of physicians based on:	Authority of physicians based on:
Specialized knowledge	Control of knowledge
Technical skills	Limited entry into profession
Professional ethics	Sovereignty over system
Physicians are seen as altruistic healers	Physicians act as self-interested entrepreneurs
Physicians adopt a paternalistic approach to patients	Physicians face conflicting loyalties in their dealings with patients
Physicians act as unbiased agents for their patients	Physicians act as imperfect agents for their patients

[a]See Parsons 1951, 1975,
[b]See Freidson 1970

medical care. The power of the medical profession has been used to support and protect the role of the individual physician as self-interested entrepreneur. By creating and maintaining a system that approached medical care as a purely market commodity, physicians were able to establish their right to charge a separate fee for each service they provided, and to base that fee on whatever the market would bear. Thus, in making medical decisions, physicians were simultaneously looking out for the needs of the patient and for their own financial interests. Both the perceived quality of care and the physician's income went up as the physician did more for the patient. This system of dual loyalties can place the physician in the role of an imperfect agent when making or recommending treatment decisions on the patient's behalf (Freidson 1970).

These alternative views of the medical profession, as agents of reason or as agents of power, are described in Table 1.1.

As we proceed in our examination of health care in the United States we will find that neither view offers a totally accurate view of the American medical profession. Medicine in this country has instead developed as a blending of the two models. For much of the last century, our health care system and the medical profession's authority over it was stable and non-controversial. It has only been since 1970, as the rising cost of health care and the growing number of uninsured Americans have commanded more attention in the public agenda, that we have seen a full examination of the effects of approaching medical care as a market commodity and sanctioning the use of medical knowledge as a source of political and economic power. These two policies have had profound impacts on the development of our health care system, and have differentiated our system from those of other industrialized countries.

Concept 1.1

Two policies established early in the twentieth century had major effects on our system of care and contributed to our current problems:

- Approaching medical care as a market commodity
- Granting sovereignty to the medical profession over the organization and financing of medical care

---

The Rising Cost of Health Care in America

In 1970, people in the United States spent a total of $73 billion, or an average of $341 per person per year, on all types of health care combined. The total national expenditure on health care represented 7.1% of the gross domestic product (GDP). At that time people talked about a national health care expenditure of 7% of GDP as representing a "crisis" that needed to be addressed urgently.

In 1998, we as a country spent $1.149 trillion on health care, or about $4094 per person. This level of expenditure represented 13.5% of GDP, nearly twice the amount of GDP apportioned to health care just 28 years earlier. After a recent pause in the growth of national expenditures for health care, current indicators point to continued escalation in the share of GDP we spend on health care. Recent government figures point to health care consuming 16.2% of GDP by 2008 (data from U.S. Health Care Financing Administration).

Where does all this money for health care come from and where does it go? Figures 1.1 and 1.2 show the sources of the money that pays for health care and the principal categories of national health care expenditures.

To get a better sense of what these data mean it is useful to compare our country to other developed countries in the world. The Organization for Economic Cooperation and Development (OECD) compiles economic and other statistics from 29 of the world's leading developed countries. Table 1.2 shows national expenditures on health care for a selection of OECD countries. In 1998 the U.S. reported that it spent 13.6% of GDP on health care. This was by far the highest expenditure in the world. The second biggest expenditure was by Germany, at 10.6%.

Why are we so concerned about how much we spend on health care? Despite the rise in the percentage of GDP allocated to health care, our economy has been thriving for years. What's the harm of all this? The answer to this question becomes clear when we consider two factors: The effect on businesses and the economy, and the effect on government.

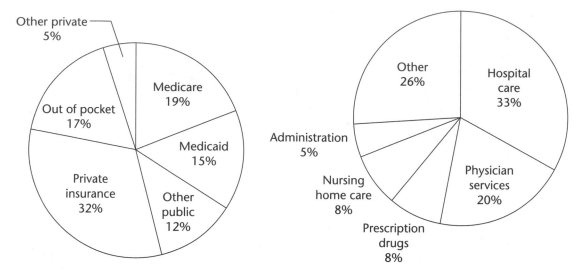

Figure 1.1 U.S. Health Care Spending, 1998: Where It Came From

Source: U.S. Health Care Financing Administration (HCFA)

Figure 1.2 U.S. Health Care Spending, 1998: Where It Went

Source: HCFA

Table 1.2   National Health Care Expenses for Selected OECD Countries, 1998

Country	Percent of GDP
United Kingdom	6.7
Japan	7.6
Sweden	8.4
Canada	9.5
France	9.6
Switzerland	10.4
Germany	10.6
United States	13.6

Source: OECD

Effect on Businesses and the U.S. Economy

Figure 1.3 shows the path health care expenditures will take if current government projections through 2008 are accurate, and the growth in health care continues at the average rate of increase seen in the last 30 years. If the pattern of growth continues, by the year 2030 nearly 25% of the entire national economy will be spent on health care. This investment in health care will be at the expense of other sectors of the economy such as educa-

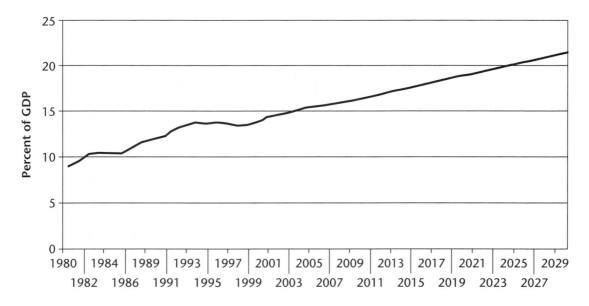

Figure 1.3 U.S. Health Care Expenditures as Percentage of GDP, 1980–1998 (Actual) and 1999–2030 (Projected)
Source: HCFA

tion and national infrastructure. We will have less money available for schools, less available for roads and other forms of transportation, and less money for investing in the capital and technology necessary for continued expansion of the economy. In addition, the high costs faced by American employers in providing health care for their workers will place U.S. companies at a severe competitive disadvantage vis-à-vis foreign companies that don't face such extreme health care costs.

Effect on Government

Beyond the potentially devastating effect on American businesses, health care expenditures in this range of GDP will have severe consequences for government as well. Recall from Figure 1.1 that governments at all levels— federal, state, and local—are responsible for a combined 46% of all health care expenditures. Governments rely on taxation to obtain revenue. Unless tax rates change, tax revenues generally rise at the same rate as GDP. However, the history of health care in this country is that the cost of care rises more rapidly than GDP. (This is especially true during times of recession, when health care costs have historically continued to rise even in the face of a shrinking economy.) This pattern of increases in health care expenditures that outpace growth in the GDP is what leads to a rising percentage of GDP dedicated to health care.

> ## Concept 1.2
>
> If the rising cost of health care as a percentage of GDP is not slowed, the impacts on our economy will be substantial:
>
> • Investment in other sectors of the economy will shrink.
>
> • American businesses will be at a competitive disadvantage with foreign competitors.
>
> • Federal, state, and local governments will have to either raise taxes or go increasingly in debt.

Now consider the effect on governments of health care expenditures rising faster than the GDP, and therefore faster than tax revenues. Forty-six percent of the rise in health care costs over the rise in GDP will have to come from government sources. *For every dollar that health care costs go up faster than GDP, government sources will pay 46¢.* This is an important concept to understand.

How will government come up with the money to pay for this rise, given that tax revenues increase only as fast as GDP increases? There will be two options: either increase tax rates to cover the increased cost of care, or borrow the needed money, thus adding to government debt. Neither choice is palatable to politicians or the American public. Either would have a severe, long-term, destabilizing effect on the American economy. Governments will face a serious dilemma if a solution to the rising cost of health care is not found.

The Growing Number of Uninsured Americans

The rising cost of health care in this country has brought with it a second problem of growing proportions. Health care has become so expensive that fewer and fewer people can afford basic health insurance. In 1999, 42.6 million people in this country had no health insurance, including more than 10 million children. One person in six was unable to afford insurance. Six states, including California and Texas, had more than one in five residents without insurance. For families who earned less than $25,000, one person in four was without insurance, even after taking into account government-financed insurance through the Medicaid program for the poor (data from U.S. Census Bureau).

During most of the twentieth century, little attention was paid to the issue of the uninsured. Most doctors would take care of some poor and uninsured patients for free. Doctors would often include a number of these charity cases in their practice, in a manner similar to lawyers taking certain cases pro bono. The ethics of the profession expected doctors to provide this type of care. With the rising cost of medical care, and with the advent in the 1960s of government programs to pay for care, the charity patient tradition has largely been abandoned by American physicians.

Who are the uninsured? It is easy to think of them as the chronically poor who don't work and who rely on government welfare for their existence. This picture could not be farther from the truth. The unemployed and the homeless make up only a small part of the uninsured. Seventy-five percent of adults between 18 and 65 without health insurance in 1999 worked either part-time or full-time during the year. They are the workers in low-wage jobs, often in small companies that don't offer health insurance to their workers. For workers earning $7 per hour or less in 1996, 43% had health insurance available as a fringe benefit from their work; for those earning more than $15 per hour, 93% had health insurance available (Cooper and Schone 1997). Roughly two-thirds of people who work for firms with 100 or more employees receive health insurance as a fringe benefit. For those working in firms with 25 or fewer employees, fewer than one-third receive health insurance. Next time you are in a fast-food restaurant, look around at the workers there. There is a good chance that the people preparing and serving your food do not receive health insurance, and that the manager who supervises them does.

The Health of Our Society—What Do We Get for Our Money?

We pay more for health insurance than any other country, both per capita and as a percentage of GDP. Yet, we are the only developed country that leaves health insurance to the market, and as a result are the only country facing the problem of the uninsured. What do we get for all the money we spend? One would hope that all that health care would make our society one of the healthiest in the world. Nothing could be farther from the truth. In comparing ourselves to other developed countries, we lag far behind in most of the broad indices that measure the overall state of the health of a society.

Infant mortality is one of the most common indicators used to gauge the health of a nation. Infant mortality measures the following statistic: Out of 1000 babies born alive, how many will die before their first birthday? Infant mortality for selected OECD countries is shown in Table 1.3, along with the percentage of GDP each country spends on health care. In 1996, the last year in which all OECD countries reported data, the United States reported an infant mortality rate of 7.8 deaths per 1000 live births. This placed us 25th out of the 29 OECD countries, worse off than Greece and Portugal. Only Hungary, Mexico, Poland, and Turkey reported worse infant mortality than the United States.

It should be apparent that there is little relation between how much a country spends on health care and the health of that society, as measured by infant mortality. Despite our spending nearly twice as much as Japan, babies in the United States still die at more than twice the rate of babies in Japan.

Another common health index is life expectancy. Life expectancy can be measured in two ways:

- Life expectancy at birth
- Age-adjusted life expectancy (How long, on average, can a person who is a certain age today expect to live?)

Life expectancy, like infant mortality, is often used to measure the health of a society. It is usually reported separately for men and women, since biological differences between the sexes historically give women an advantage over men in longevity. How does the United States compare to other developed countries in this statistic? The answer is shown in Table 1.4.

In 1998, male babies born in the United States could expect to live, on average, 73.9 years, and girls born the same year could expect to live 79.4 years. Out of the 23 OECD countries who reported data for 1998, we ranked 15th for male life expectancy and 16th for females. Again, babies born in Greece can expect to live longer than those born in the United States.

In addition to measuring life expectancy at birth, additional information about the health of a society can be obtained by looking at age-specific life expectancy: For adults who have attained a certain age, how many additional years can they expect to live on average? Table 1.5 compares the United States with four other developed countries: France, Japan, Sweden, and the United Kingdom. It compares life expectancy in these countries at ages 40, 60, and 80. Data for ages 40 and 60 are from 1997, and are from the OECD. Data for age 80 are not reported by OECD and are available only for 1987 (Manton and Vaupel 1995).

The United States is fifth out of these five countries in life expectancy at birth. At age 40 we are fifth in life expectancy only for men; for women we are fourth. At age 60 we are fourth out of five for both men and women. At age 80, however, the United States has the best life expectancy of all five countries. In 1987, 80-year-old men in the United States lived ten months longer than those in the United Kingdom and one month longer than those in Japan. Eighty-year-old women lived twelve months longer than those in the United Kingdom and six months longer than those in Japan.

It appears that the principal health benefit our society enjoys as a result of our heavy investment in health care is greater life expectancy for our 80-

Table 1.3   1996 Infant Mortality for Selected OECD Countries, 1996

Country	Percent of GDP Spent on Health Care	Infant Mortality[a]
Japan	7.2	3.8
Sweden	8.6	4.0
Switzerland	10.2	4.7
France	9.8	4.8
Germany	10.5	5.0
Canada	9.2	6.0
United Kingdom	6.9	6.1
Greece	6.8	7.3
United States	13.6	7.8

[a] Infant deaths per 1000 live births
Source: OECD

Table 1.4   Life Expectancy at Birth for Selected OECD Countries, 1998

Country	Male Life Expectancy (years)	Female Life Expectancy (years)
Japan	77.2	84.0
Sweden	76.9	81.9
Switzerland	76.5	82.2
France	74.6	82.5
Germany	74.5	80.5
Canada	75.8	81.4
United Kingdom	74.6	79.7
Greece	75.3	80.5
United States	73.9	79.4

Source: OECD

year-olds. This is understandable, since the common causes of death for people in these age groups—heart attacks, cancer, and strokes—are often amenable to high-tech treatment. Because we have more health care technology available than any other country, it stands to reason that our oldest citizens should fare better than their counterparts in countries that invest less than we do in high-tech health care. However, at ages younger than 80 there seems to be little relationship between the amount we spend on health care and the health of our population.

Table 1.5   Life Expectancy in Additional Years at Ages 40, 60, and 80
for Selected OECD Countries

Country	Men Age 40	Women Age 40	Men Age 60	Women Age 60	Men Age 80	Women Age 80
France	36.7	43.5	20.0	25.2	6.7	8.6
Japan	38.6	44.8	20.9	26.1	6.9	8.5
Sweden	38.1	42.7	20.1	24.2	6.5	8.3
United Kingdom	36.4	40.8	18.8	22.6	6.2	8.1
United States	36.2	40.9	19.4	23.1	7.0	9.1

[a]Data for ages 40 and 60 are from the OECD, and are for 1997.
[b]Data for age 80 are from Manton and Vaupel 1995, and are for 1987.

As the above data suggest, it is difficult to compare the quality of national health systems when different measures of quality give such disparate rankings. In order to reconcile some of these differences the World Health Organization has created a single measure of the overall quality of a nation's health system. This measure of overall health system attainment combines the following three measures:

1. Disability-adjusted life expectancy
2. Degree of equality within the system
3. Level of financing of the system

Using this combined measure, the United States ranked 15th in the world, slightly ahead of Spain and Greece (World Health Report 2000).

Concept 1.3

The United States spends more on health care than any other country in the world. Despite this high level of expenditure, we have one of the lowest levels of overall health of any developed country. The only measure of health in which our country excels is the additional number of years an 80-year-old person can expect to live.

What Determines the Overall Health of a Society?

It should by now be clear that, at the level of the society, health care and health are not the same thing. Using the above indicators, there is little if any correlation between the amount spent on health care and the health of a society. As the country spending by far the most, we still have health indices close to the worst. The only exception is in the survival of our 80-year-olds, and this difference is relatively small.

Rather than the amount of money spent on health care, other factors largely determine the overall health of a society. Principal among these is overall standard of living, typically measured by per capita income and the average level of education in a society. Victor Fuchs, one of the founders of the study of health economics, has repeatedly emphasized this relationship.

> *The basic finding is the following: when the state of medical science and other health-determining variables are held constant, the marginal contribution of medical care to health is very small in modern nations. . . . For most of man's history, [per capita] income has been the primary determinant of health and life expectancy—the major explanation for differences in health among nations and among groups within a nation. (Fuchs 1986, pp. 274–276)*

An excellent example of the ways in which social class and standard of living affect health independently from health care is seen in Great Britain.

Concept 1.4

Among developed countries, there is little correlation between the amount a country spends on health care and the overall level of health of that country. The health of a society has more to do with the level of education and income than it does with health care.

The Whitehall study looked at the health of people working in the British Civil Service (Marmot and Theorell 1988). Britain has had universal health coverage and a nationalized health system since World War II, so all members of the Civil Service have access to basically the same level of health care. Thus differences in health care cannot explain differences in health.

The study found a clear correlation between income (and therefore education) and health. There was a threefold difference in mortality between the highest and the lowest ranks of the Civil Service. Even at the upper ranks, the higher on the scale a worker was, the lower the mortality he or she faced. This was true even though all subjects of the study worked in office jobs, were regularly employed, came from a relatively uniform ethnic background, and lived and worked in greater London.

These data should not be taken to mean that there has been no improvement in overall health in the face of the growing cost of health care in this country. Quite the contrary: data from the last 40 years show dramatic increases in health. In 1960, when the United States spent 5.2% of GDP on health care, infant mortality was at the level of 26 deaths per 1000 live births; now it is 7.8. Male life expectancy was 66.6 years in 1960 and is now 72.7. Female life expectancy went from 73.1 to 79.4 years. It is simply that despite these improvements in overall health, we still lag far behind other developed countries.

There is substantial evidence suggesting that improvements in the level of health in this country may be due more to lifestyle changes than to improvements in health care. Our decreased rate of heart disease, for example, appears to be related more to improved diet and exercise than to improvements in drugs or surgical treatments (Burke et al. 1991).

Victor Fuchs provides an example of the importance of lifestyle in his book, *Who Shall Live*. He cites data for Nevada and Utah, two states with roughly comparable populations in terms of ethnic background, socioeconomic status, education, climate, and availability of medical care. In the 1960s, infant mortality in Nevada was 40% higher than in Utah, and life expectancy in Nevada was 40–50% lower than in Utah. If income, education, and medical care cannot explain these differences, what can?

Cigarette and alcohol consumption are markedly lower in Utah, due largely to the influence of the Mormon Church. Correspondingly, death rates from cirrhosis of the liver and lung cancer are two to three times higher in Nevada than in Utah. Lifestyle factors in Nevada and Utah, rather than medical care, seem to have explained the different levels of health in the two states.

It appears that further increasing expenditures for health care cannot be expected to result in substantial improvements in the overall health of American society. Nonetheless there is a strong social movement to provide increased access for the uninsured. Providing health insurance to the one-sixth of our society that is uninsured will add substantially to the overall cost of health care.

There is also, however, an equally forceful movement to hold down the cost of medical care. Thus we face two powerful, opposing forces—the need to expand access to health care and the need to hold down costs of care. Despite years of discussion and debate we don't seem to be able to find a solution to this dilemma. The problems of health care access and cost involve powerful yet often conflicting forces. To understand why we have this difficulty, and to understand the importance of institutional factors in American health care, Chapter 2 compares of health care in Canada and the United States.

ON-LINE DATA SOURCES

Data about national health care expenditures in the U.S. are available from the
United States Health Care Financing Administration (HCFA) at www.hcfa.gov
Throughout this book I make reference to the Health Care Financing Administration (HCFA), the agency within the federal government that is responsible for most of the major health programs. While this book was in press the Bush administration changed the name of the agency to the Centers for Medicare and Medicaid Services (CMS). At the time the book went to the printer the internet address for the agency was still www.hcfa.gov.

Data about the number of uninsured are available from the U.S. Census Bureau at
www.census.gov.

Data about comparative national health statistics are available from the Organization for Economic Cooperation and Development (OECD) at www.oecd.org.

The World Health Report 2000 is published by the World Health Organization and
is available at www.who.org.

REFERENCES

Bowman JG. Standard of Efficiency. *Bulletin of the American College of Surgeons*. 1918; III(3):1.

Burke GL, Sprafka JM, Folsom AR et al. Trends in Serum Cholesterol Levels from 1980 to 1987. *New England Journal of Medicine*. 1991; 324: 941–46.

Cooper PE, Schone BS. More Offers, Fewer Takers for Employment-Based Health Insurance: 1987 and 1996. *Health Affairs*. 1997; 16(6):142–48.

Flexner A. *Medical Education in the United States and Canada*. New York: Carnegie Foundation for the Advancement of Teaching, 1910.

Freidson E. *Profession of Medicine: A Study of the Sociology of Applied Knowledge*. New York: Dodd, Mead, 1970.

Fuchs, VR. *Who Shall Live*. New York: Basic Books, 1983.

Fuchs VR. *The Health Economy*. Cambridge, Mass.: Harvard University Press, 1986.

Manton KG, Vaupel JW. Survival After the Age of 80 in the United States, Sweden, France, England, and Japan. *New England Journal of Medicine*. 1995; 333:1232–35.

Marmot MG, Theorell T. Social Class and Cardiovascular Disease: The Contribution of Work. *International Journal of Health Services*. 1988; 18:659–74.

Parsons, *The Social System*. New York: Free Press, 1951, pp. 428–79.

Parsons, The Sick Role and the Role of the Physician Revisited. *Millbank Memorial Fund Quarterly*. 1975; 53:257.

Reinhardt UE, Relman AS. Debating For-Profit Health Care and the Ethics of Physicians. *Health Affairs*. 1986; 5(2):5–31.

Sade, RM. Medical Care as a Right: A Refutation. *New England Journal of Medicine*. 1971; 285:1288–92.

Starr P. The *Social Transformation of American Medicine*. New York: Basic Books, 1982.

Health Care in America as a Reflection of Underlying Cultural Values and Institutions

Key Concepts

- A monopsony is an economic system that has a single payer for a set of goods or services. The Canadian health care system is an example of a government monopsony in health care, sometimes called a single-payer system.
- The Canadian health care system is based on the following principles of social policy:

    Health care is a basic right of all Canadians.

    The power of the medical profession is limited by its social obligation.

    There is one standard of health care for all Canadians.

    The government retains monopsony power over the payment for health care (i.e., Canada's is a single-payer system)

- The U.S. health care system is based on the following principles of social policy:

    Health care is a market commodity to be distributed according to ability to pay.

    Power over the organization and delivery of health care has historically been concentrated in the medical profession.

    There is no uniform standard of care. The quality of care received often reflects the ability to pay.

    Government has historically had relatively little role in guiding our system of health care.

- In the United States, the value we as a society place on technology and technological advances encourages the development and use of high-tech medical treatments, even when the added benefit of these treatments is small compared to their cost.
- In the United States, the institution of medical malpractice represents a combination of the following factors:

    A poor outcome for the patient

    A substantial level of disability as a result

A poor interpersonal relationship between the patient and the physician

Only in rare circumstances actual physician negligence

- Cultural institutions unique to the United States have helped create a health care system that is the most expensive in the world while excluding more people from care than any developed country. Any attempt to reform the system to address these problems must consider the institutions that led to the problems in the first place.

The Cultural Basis of Health Care Delivery: Comparing the United States and Canada

The organization of medicine is not a thing apart which can be subjected to study in isolation. It is an aspect of culture, whose arrangements are inseparable from the general organization of society. (Walton H. Hamilton, 1932)

This statement, made more than 70 years ago, still rings true in our examination of health care in America in the twenty-first century. To understand a nation's health care system, it is important first to understand the social and cultural norms and values around which that nation is organized.

In order to appreciate fully how the health care system in the United States reflects our unique American value system, we can look to our neighbors to the north. Using Canada and its health care system as a mirror, we see how differences in the organization of health care in our two countries reflect differences in the basic institutions around which our systems are organized.

Lipset (1990, p. 2) describes the fundamental similarities and differences between United States and Canadian societies. He reminds us of the cultural differences that arose from the time of the American Revolution:

The very organizing principles that frame these nations, the central cores around which institutions and events were to accommodate, were different. One was Whig and classically liberal or libertarian—doctrines that emphasize distrust of the state, egalitarianism, and populism. . . . The other was Tory and conservative in the British and European sense—accepting of the need for a strong state, for respect for authority, for deference.

In the United States, schoolchildren study the Declaration of Independence and learn that our society is organized around the principles of "life, liberty, and the pursuit of happiness." Canadian children also learn about the founding principles of their country. In the British North America Act, which created the Dominion of Canada, they find that the role of the Canadian government is to ensure "peace, order, and good government."

> *The Canadian Charter of Rights and Freedoms is not the American Bill of Rights. It preserves the principle of parliamentary supremacy and places less emphasis on individual, as distinct from group, rights than does the American document. (Lipset 1990, p. 3)*

Since the American Revolution, the United States has been a country that puts primacy on the rights of individuals. Social justice is most often defined in terms of the individual. In the United States, conflicts between individual and group needs tend to be resolved in favor of the individual. Canada, on the other hand, has a strong social democratic tradition, a tradition of redistribution so as to maximize the common good. Canadians have come to accept and expect social policies that embody this individual:group relationship. In Canada, conflicts between individual and group rights tend to be resolved in favor of the common good. These differences between United States and Canadian society are summarized in Table 2.1.

Table 2.1   Cultural Differences Between the United States and Canada

United States	Canada
Distrust of central government	Accepting the need for strong
central government	
"Life, liberty, and the pursuit of happiness"	"Peace, order, and good government"
Justice often defined in terms of	Justice often defined so as to
what is good for the individual	maximize the common good

To see how these cultural differences are reflected in health care systems, we first examine the history of Canadian health care.

The Historical Development of the Canadian Health Care System

The British North America Act of 1867 created the Dominion of Canada. In it, responsibility for managing medical care delivery was explicitly vested in the provinces rather than the central government. This separation of powers for health care issues remains in place today.

Canada took a serious look at establishing a national system of health care following World War I. At that time, several provinces granted to municipalities the statutory authority to become directly involved in the provision of medical care. During the Great Depression, these "municipal doctor" plans, in which local governments hired doctors to provide care to area residents, became an increasingly important source of medical care. This was especially true in the rural, agricultural provinces (Meilicke and Storch 1980).

In 1943, the report of a governmental Economic Advisory Committee recommended that a national program of medical insurance be established. It was to have been part of a larger social insurance program also covering unemployment insurance and old age security. Despite the support of both the Canadian Medical Association and the Canadian Hospital Council, the program failed to become law, the result principally of the failure to achieve a financing mechanism that adequately preserved perceptions of provincial autonomy.

As a largely rural province with a widely scattered population especially hard-hit by the depression, Saskatchewan faced a particularly pressing need for governmental support of medical care. In 1944, Saskatchewan elected a populist government by giving a large legislative majority to the Cooperative Commonwealth Federation (CCF). In the face of the earlier defeat of the proposed national health care program, one of the first priorities for the CCF in Saskatchewan was to bring provincial government support to the financing of hospital care. The Saskatchewan Hospital Services Plan was passed in 1946, establishing a universal, compulsory hospital care insurance system. The program did not cover physicians' fees.

Despite increased rates of hospital utilization and costs in excess of initial estimates, the Saskatchewan plan maintained popular support. By 1950, three other provinces had established similar hospital insurance programs. It was only a matter of time before the others would follow. In 1957 the Hospital Services and Diagnostic Services Act was adopted by the federal government of Canada, establishing a national program of universal, compulsory hospital insurance, based on the Saskatchewan model. The program established three important principles:

1. Shared financing between the federal and the provincial governments that partially compensated for economic inequities between provinces
2. Provincial administration of the plan
3. Federally established minimum standards of participation

Saskatchewan again took action that was to have national impact. Having previously financed hospital care solely from provincial funds, the sudden addition of federal hospital funds enabled the CCF government to extend its medical insurance program to include physician care. In 1962 it established the Saskatchewan Medical Care Insurance Plan, creating a universal, compulsory medical care system, with the provincial government maintaining a monopsony over the purchase of all medical care. (A monopoly is an economic system with only one provider of a good; a monopsony is a system with a single payer for a good.) It was financed by a compulsory enrollment premium for all provincial residents. The plan maintained the fee-for-service method of paying physicians but established the principle that physicians must accept payment from the plan as payment in full (i.e., the physician was not allowed to bill the patient for any additional amount).

Concept 2.1

A monopsony is an economic system that has a single payer for a set of goods or services. The Canadian health care system is an example of a government monopsony in health care, sometimes called a single-payer system.

The concept of government monopsony was stridently opposed by the Canadian Medical Association, its Saskatchewan division, and by the American Medical Association (AMA) south of the border. (The role of the American Medical Association in actively opposing national health insurance in Canada is seldom fully appreciated.) However, the Saskatchewan plan was enacted over the objections of the medical profession.

On July 1, 1962, physicians in the Saskatchewan Medical Association went on strike, refusing to participate in the plan. Leaders of the association contended that "the preservation of the basic freedoms and democratic rights of the individual is necessary to insure medical services to the people of Saskatchewan" (Taylor 1987, p. 278). Saskatchewan physicians were seen as the shock troops of the medical profession, fighting the battle against governmentally imposed medical insurance on behalf of the entire Canadian medical profession. They received strong support from the AMA in the United States, which was adamantly opposed to the plan. The AMA attempted to convey a sense of crisis to the doctors and public in Saskatchewan.

Although the strike had some support within Saskatchewan, it received little support from the rest of Canada. To many people the striking physicians were seen not as altruistic professionals but as lawbreakers.

By July 23, a little more than three weeks after the strike had begun, the medical profession and the government reached a compromise, and the strike was called off. The Saskatchewan Agreement created a role for private insurance companies as fiscal intermediaries, allowing doctors to bill an insurance company for their services with the insurance company being reimbursed by the government. In return physicians agreed to accept plan payment as payment in full. In addition the Saskatchewan government promised not to establish a salaried government medical service.

In 1964, the Royal Commission on Health Services, established by the federal government to study the issue of national health insurance, recommended that Canada establish a national program of medical care similar to Saskatchewan's (Royal Commission on Health Services 1964). Its goal was to make care "available to all our residents without hindrance of any kind." It proposed federal financial assistance for provincially administered programs. Initial response to the report was mixed. Several provinces opposed further extension of government authority over health care, supporting instead a market-based program of insurance subsidies for low-income individuals and families, as had been proposed by the Canadian Medical Association.

The Liberal Party in Canada had first made a commitment to a program of national health insurance as early as 1919. In 1965 the Liberals came to power on a widely supported platform that included establishing a national system of medical care. Under the leadership of Lester Pearson, it pushed for such a program. In contrast to the legislative system in the United States, in a parliamentary government such as Canada's the prime minister is able to exert considerable influence over the legislative process. Pearson pursued and, despite the opposition of several provinces, in December 1966 achieved passage of the National Medicare program. Provincial participation was to be voluntary; participation, if adopted by the provinces, would result in federal payment of approximately half the cost of the program. For a provincial program to qualify it had to be comprehensive, universal, publicly administered, and portable across provinces. (A fifth principle of accessibility was added later.)

The Canadian Medicare program went into effect in 1968. The lure of a 50% federal subsidy proved to be powerful. By 1971 all 10 provinces had qualifying programs, creating on a national scale the same government monopsony over the purchase of medical care that had been established in Saskatchewan. The private market for medical insurance in Canada was effectively eliminated.

The Canadian Medicare program did not adopt a specific model for the organization or delivery of care. It was solely a financing mechanism, leaving the delivery of care to physicians and the provinces. The federal government simply agreed to reimburse 50% of the cost of care to any province that created a plan meeting the guiding principles.

This time it was doctors in the province of Quebec who went on strike in opposition to the plan. Quebec had two separate provincial medical associations: one for general practitioners and one for specialists. The association of specialists wanted its members to be able to opt out of the plan on a case-by-case basis, billing the patient directly and allowing the patient to seek reimbursement from Medicare. (Those familiar with the U.S. Medicare program, discussed in Chapter 5, will note that the payment mechanism sought by the specialists in Quebec was precisely the mechanism adopted by the United States program only a few years earlier. The influence of the AMA on Canadian physicians' opposition to Canadian Medicare is clear.)

The specialists voted to strike rather than participate in Medicare. In early October 1970, they held a large rally in opposition to the plan. The leaders of the specialists spoke at that rally and criticized Medicare as a "threat to liberty, freedom, and quality of care." The executive vice president of the AMA also spoke at this rally. He supported the strike and assured any specialists who chose to do so that they could move south and establish their practice in the United States.

Rene Levesque, at that time leader of Le Parti Québécois and later to become premier of Quebec, publicly criticized the physicians' strike. In doing so he stated the following principle of Canadian society:

> Organized medicine derives its power from the state, and the fact that the state has granted it a monopoly on such an indispensable service involves the responsibility to make that service available. (quoted in Taylor 1987, p. 404)

Despite government opposition the specialists did go on strike on October 8. They refused to provide any care except for emergency cases. The Canadian press voiced a common criticism of the striking doctors, characterizing them as "operating in a social vacuum." Pierre Trudeau, the prime minister of Canada, was explicit in his condemnation: "Those who would defy the law and ignore the opportunities available to them to right their wrongs, and satisfy their claims, will receive no hearing from this government. We shall ensure that the laws are respected" (quoted in Taylor 1987, p. 409).

On October 10 the labor minister of Quebec was kidnapped and later murdered by radical separatists. Amidst concerns of potential civil insurrection, the specialists called off their strike without gaining any of their demands. On November 1 Quebec Medicare began without incident, with full participation of the specialists.

Following an initial leveling of medical care costs in the period immediately following enactment of Medicare, rapid increases in the mid-1970s led to a growing concern that the costs of the program were unacceptably high and rising. The share of Canadian GDP going to health care began to rise in ways similar to the rise seen in the United States. The federal government of Canada needed to make future medical care costs more predictable, and the provinces wanted more direct control of financing. Accordingly, in 1977 a new arrangement was negotiated. In exchange for transferring a portion of its taxing authority to the provinces, the federal government's share of program costs was reduced from 50% to approximately 25%. In addition, future increases in the federal contribution would be limited to actual increases in the GDP. Under the new formula, 100% of new costs exceeding the corresponding population/GDP increase would be borne by the provinces. The provinces went from being responsible for only 50 cents of every extra dollar spent on health care to facing responsibility for 100 cents on the dollar. This limitation had a powerful effect, leading to more stringent efforts at cost control throughout Canada. There followed several years of stability of medical care costs as a percentage of GDP. It was largely in this period that the gap between Canada and the United States in percentage of GDP going to health care developed.

An important modification to the original Medicare program was passed in 1984. Even though Medicare created a government monopsony on the purchase of medical care, many physicians continued the practice of "balance billing," charging patients a fee over and above the established Medicare payment. In the eyes of the Canadian government, balance billing was contrary to the principles of universality and accessibility. Led by the Ontario Medical Association, many physicians clung tenaciously to this last vestige of individual entrepreneurship. In response, the government passed the Canada Health Act in 1984. Although not actually outlawing balance billing, it mandated that for every dollar of balance billing that occurred in a province, the federal allocation to that province would correspondingly be reduced by a dollar.

The Ontario Medical Association, adamantly opposed to that act, organized a physicians' strike to protest the new restrictions. Its president contended that

> *today's physicians believe we have a solemn duty to preserve the professional freedom that has been handed down from generation to generation for 5000 years. It is unthinkable to us that our profession's traditions, honored through the ages without the benefit of legislation, could be struck down in a modern society that has enacted a Charter of Rights and Freedoms. (quoted in Taylor 1987, p. 460)*

Representatives of the provincial government responded:

> *When the state grants a monopoly to an exclusive group to render an indispensable service it automatically becomes involved in whether those services are available and on what terms and conditions. (quoted in Taylor 1987, p. 460)*

With little support in the media, the strike was called off after 28 days. As was the case in Saskatchewan 22 years earlier and Quebec 14 years earlier, the Ontario doctors' strike achieved neither widespread public support nor its stated goals.

Clearly the power of physicians and their professional associations is substantially limited in Canada, both by law and in the eyes of the public. Consistently, when physicians went on strike to protest the implementation of new health care initiatives, they were seen as violating their obligations to Canadian society that resulted from the authority granted them over the clinical practice of medicine.

The Organizing Principles of the Canadian Health Care System

From this examination of the Canadian health care system it is possible to identify four principles around which the system is organized.

1. *Health care is a basic right of all Canadians.* Canada has made a social commitment to the concept that health care is a right of all citizens. Based on this right the payment for health care is through taxes, with no direct connection between receiving care and paying for care.

2. *The power of the medical profession is limited by its social obligation.* The medical profession derives its monopoly authority over the practice of medicine from the state, and has a responsibility in return to participate in and cooperate with programs established by the government.

3. *There is one standard of health care for all Canadians.* All people in Canada, regardless of income or social position, receive essentially the same level of care. (One important exception to this principle is discussed below.)

4. *The government retains monopsony power over the payment for health care* (i.e., Canada's is a single-payer system). The success of the program depends on the monopsony power of the state. No other purchasers of health care (i.e., private insurance companies) are allowed.

Concept 2.2

The Canadian health care system is based on the following principles of social policy:

1. Health care is a basic right of all Canadians.
2. The power of the medical profession is limited by its social obligation.
3. There is one standard of health care for all Canadians.
4. The government retains monopsony power over the payment for health care (i.e., Canada's is a single-payer system).

Based on these principles, Canada has maintained its level of national expenditure for health care at between 9% and 10% of GDP, while the United States spends nearly 14% of GDP. How is it that Canada has been able to keep its expenditures so low relative to those in the United States?

Most of the provinces have instituted a series of fiscal policies ensuring that rises in health care expenditures parallel rises in GDP. These policies include

- A yearly, global budget for physician fees, with fee levels negotiated between the government and doctors so as to stay within the budget
- Fixed annual budgets for all hospitals
- Government requirements that all capital expenditures for new hospital facilities and new technology (such as magnetic resonance imaging [MRI] machines) be separately approved and financed

Although these fiscal policies have been successful in holding down the cost of the system, they have had an important consequence for Canadians seeking care: queuing. Queuing refers to the need for many patients to go on a waiting list before receiving certain types of tests or treatments. Once referred by their physician, people often have to wait many months before obtaining an MRI or other types of tests that rely on expensive technology. The policy of holding down expenditures for these technologies has resulted in their short supply relative to the demand for them. Similarly, patients referred for surgical procedures such as heart bypass, cataract removal, or hip replacement (all elective procedures that do not carry a major risk if delayed) may be scheduled for surgery months in the future. Generally, care is taken to put patients in urgent need of these procedures at the front of the line, although budgetary problems that developed in the 1990s opened this principle to question.

Despite the spending controls that were part of the system, the cost of medical care in Canada continued to escalate throughout the 1980s. Faced with mounting economic problems at both the federal and provincial level, many of the provincial plans began to experience severe shortages of both personnel and facilities in the mid-1990s. Newspaper and television reports documented increasing waits for services, often including services such as emergency room care or biopsies of possibly cancerous breast lumps. Public support for the health care system declined substantially; whereas 61% of the population rated the system as excellent in 1991, only 24% rated it as excellent in 1999 (Iglehart 2000).

The principle behind queuing for care in Canada is that scarce health care resources are allocated first to those in the greatest need, measured in terms of the risk to their life or health. Those with lesser need must simply wait their turn. Here is where the Canadian system of providing one level of care for all people breaks down somewhat. Nearly 90% of all Canadians live within 100 miles of the United States border. Those waiting in the queue for an elective test or procedure have the option of simply traveling to the United States (where health care is available as a market commodity) and paying cash to obtain the test or procedure. Given the expense involved, this option is realistically available only to the wealthiest Canadians. Thus, to a certain extent, Canada operates a two-tiered system. One tier is available to every Canadian, although it frequently results in queuing for expensive tests and procedures. The second tier is available without queuing to those few who can afford to travel to the United States and pay out of pocket.

The Organizing Principles of the United States Health Care System

The principles around which the United States health care system is organized stand in sharp contrast to those of the Canadian system. They reflect our society's view of the importance of the rights of the individual and of our general distrust of government programs.

1. *Health care is a market commodity to be distributed according to ability to pay.* Other than basic emergency services, there is no acknowledged right to health care for those under 65 years of age. (The federal Medicare program, discussed in Chapter 5, provides health coverage for all people 65 years or older who qualify for Social Security.) As discussed in Chapter 1, this principle reflects a decision made during the early part of the twentieth century, and continues to guide the distribution of access to care.

2. *Power over the organization and delivery of health care has historically been concentrated in the medical profession.* Since the Flexner report, both state and federal governments have relied on the medical profession to establish standards of education and licensure, guide medical ethics, define financing mechanisms for care, and control the ways in which hospitals are utilized.

3. *There is no uniform standard of care.* The quality of care received often reflects the ability to pay. Ours has evolved into a multitiered health care system, with differing levels of quality at different tiers. Differences in quality reflect both differences in the training and skills of the physician and differences in access to care.

4. *Government has historically had relatively little role in guiding our system of health care.* Although government's role has been increasing in recent years due to its increasing role in paying for care, throughout most of the twentieth century there was little in the way of government policy or programs intended to establish a national system of either providing or paying for care.

It should by now be clear that the system of care in the United States is fundamentally different from that in Canada, reflecting fundamental cul-

---

Concept 2.3

The United States health care system is based on the following principles of social policy:

1. Health care is a market commodity to be distributed according to ability to pay.
2. Power over the organization and delivery of health care has histor-ically been concentrated in the medical profession.
3. There is no uniform standard of care. The quality of care received often reflects the ability to pay.
4. Government has historically had relatively little role in guiding our system of health care.

---

tural differences between our two countries. This conclusion reinforces one of the principal messages of this text: in order to understand our health care system, it is necessary to understand the institutional forces unique to the United States that shape that system.

Cultural Institutions That Drive Health Care in the United States

The concept of an "institution" refers to the rules a society adopts that create its social, political, and economic structure. To appreciate more fully the way culturally derived institutions shape our lives, consider the following examples.

When meeting someone in this country for the first time, one typically offers a handshake. No written rules say we must; nevertheless failure to do so might be considered rude.

When eating in a restaurant while traveling away home we typically leave a tip. Even though we may never be at that restaurant again and may never again encounter our server (thus not having to worry about how good the service will be the next time we are here), we still feel obliged to leave a tip. Not to do so would be insensitive to the server.

People often discuss "the institution of marriage," its pros and cons, and the way it has changed. Here they are talking both about the formal laws that govern marriage and the social roles people fill when married.

In most circles Stanford University is seen as a well-respected academic institution. In both the written rules that govern the education it offers and the unwritten rules that govern relationships among individuals and groups, the very character of the university is created.

The U.S. Congress has often been talked about as one of the most ineffective political institutions one could imagine. In its endless rules and procedures, committees and subcommittees, it sometimes seems as though the legislative process were designed never to get anything done.

What links all these United States institutions? What do they all have in common? To understand the answer to this question is to understand one of the key driving forces behind the problems we face in health care today.

Each example above represents rules of social interaction that most people understand and take largely for granted. Douglas North (1986, pp. 3–4), a Nobel–Prize-winning economist, describes how institutions shape our social as well as our economic lives: "[Institutions] are a guide to human interaction, so that when we wish to greet friends on the street, drive an automobile, buy oranges, borrow money, form a business, bury our dead, or whatever, we know (or can learn easily) how to perform those tasks. . . . Institutions may be created, as was the United States Constitution; or they may simply evolve over time, as does the common law."

Institutions can be formal, as in written laws, codes of ethics, and prescribed procedures, or they can be informal, such as common courtesy and the strength of family ties. Many institutions have both formal and informal aspects. Consider, for example, the medical profession. As discussed above, in this country the medical profession is commonly viewed as exercising authority over the use of specialized knowledge in ways that contribute to the social good. This perception arose informally over time. The widely held view of the medical profession led to the creation of laws that formalized this role, granting the profession autonomous authority over medical education, licensure, and practice.

Institutions have four defining characteristics (Scott 1987):

- They are rules that guide behavior in certain situations.
- The rules can be formal or informal.
- Over time those rules come to be taken largely for granted.
- Disobeying the rules will invoke some sort of sanction, again either formal or informal.

In one way, institutions tend to be socially efficient. They allow us to enter into situations without having to figure out from scratch what to do every time. However, not all institutions turn out to be quite so efficient. Again quoting Douglas North (1986, p. 16): "Institutions are not necessarily or even usually created to be socially efficient; rather they, or at least the formal rules, are created to serve the interests of those with the bargaining power to devise new rules."

Where do institutions come from? The process through which institutions are created has been characterized as "profoundly political and reflect[ing] the relative power of organized interests and the actors who mobilize around them" (DiMaggio 1988). Economists, political scientists, and sociologists seem to agree that institutions often reflect, at least initially, the needs of powerful, organized interests. However, they do not change easily or quickly even in the face of a changing economic or political context. Once established, institutions limit the opportunity for further changes in social policy over the course of a nation's history. Institutions "may assume a life of their own, a life independent of the basic causal factors that led to their creation in the first place" (Krasner 1983, p. 357). This is not to say that institutions do not change; rather they change gradually, reflecting only changes in economic forces and social perceptions that persist over time.

In comparing health care in the United States and Canada we find fundamental differences in policy. We identified two key policies that differentiate health care in the United States from that in Canada and other developed countries: approaching medical care as a market commodity, and granting sovereignty to the medical profession over the organization and financing of care. In addition, we have discussed how health care in Canada is organized around improving the common good, whereas care in the United States is organized around the rights of the individual. These three differences in policy represent institutional differences that have developed out of the social and political differences between the United States and Canada. In the United States these institutions tend to push up the costs of health care while other institutional forces (for example, the American aversion to paying taxes) hold down the funds available to pay for health care. The result is that one person in six has no health insurance coverage.

Protein Deprivation, Prime Rib, and Declining Marginal Returns

To understand more fully how institutional forces affect the cost of care, let us consider a basic principle of economics: the law of declining marginal returns. To illustrate this law, I offer the following story from personal experience.

One summer I was on a backpacking trip with my son in the Wind River wilderness in Wyoming. After seven days of hiking at high altitude, during which we survived mostly on freeze-dried food, nuts, and raisins, we came out of the wilderness and went in search of a real meal. I usually don't eat much red meat, but when we walked into the restaurant in the small town near the trailhead, the aroma of prime rib of beef hit us. Having been protein deprived during our trip, my digestive system cried out for a plate of prime rib. I gave in. Never have I enjoyed a meal quite so much as I enjoyed that prime rib. I would gladly have paid $50 for it. Fortunately it only cost $11.95.

Now, while I actually stopped at one plate, for the sake of discussion let us assume a clever waiter. Seeing how much I enjoyed the first plate, he encourages me to order a second. "After all, you enjoyed the first one so much, think how much you'll enjoy the second." So I give in and order a second plate. I find that I derive substantially less enjoyment from the second than the first. While I would have paid $50 for the first plate, I wouldn't pay a penny more than $11.95 for the second.

The waiter then encourages me to order a third plate. Again I give in. While I did derive some benefit from eating the third plate, it was only a small benefit—say $1.00 worth of benefit. The waiter starts to get very pushy and brings me a fourth plate. Not wanting to hurt his feelings I begin to eat it, but part way through I get up, go into the rest room, and throw up everything.

This story seems on the surface a bit silly. What rational person would pay $11.95 for a plate of prime rib from which he only derived $1.00 worth of benefit? Even more, who would ever willingly pay for food that he knows will probably make him sick? And besides, what does this have to

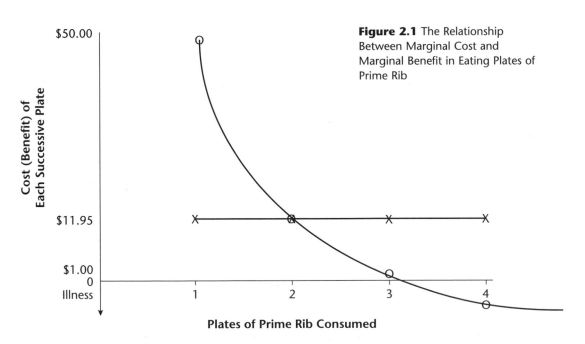

Figure 2.1 The Relationship Between Marginal Cost and Marginal Benefit in Eating Plates of Prime Rib

X = Marginal cost
O = Marginal benefit

do with health care? To understand, let us create a graph describing my folly in ordering prime rib (see Figure 2.1).

Consistent with the law of declining marginal returns, for each successive meal I order, I derive less benefit (here measured in enjoyment and willingness to pay) than from the previous meal. A person who is acting rationally would never order more than two meals. He would stop at the point where the marginal benefit equals the marginal return. This point—the intersection of the line of marginal costs and that of marginal benefits—is one definition of economic efficiency.

Let us stay with the law of declining marginal returns but move back to health care. Although the issues are quite different, the principle is the same. Figure 2.2 illustrates the effect of declining marginal returns in health care.

The Figure 2.2 graph can be used to represent decisions at the level of the individual patient and at the level of the health care system overall. For the individual patient, consider the example of a college student who falls down and twists her knee while playing recreational soccer. Her knee becomes sore and swollen. Her first decision is whether to go to the doctor for an exam, or simply wait to see what happens if she rests the knee and gives it a chance to heal. If she does go to the doctor, the first decision the

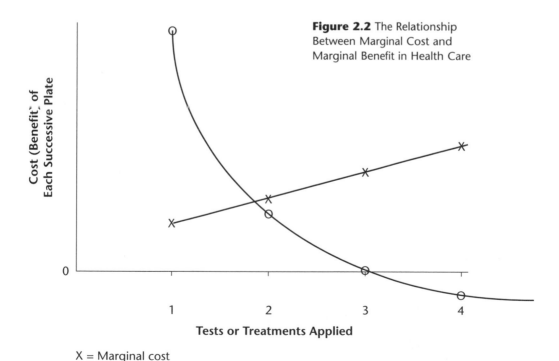

Figure 2.2 The Relationship Between Marginal Cost and Marginal Benefit in Health Care

X = Marginal cost
O = Marginal benefit

doctor may face after performing an examination is whether to X–ray the knee to see if it is broken. (While it is unlikely an injury of this type will break a bone, it is a possibility.) Assuming the physical examination performed by the doctor shows no clear evidence of a torn ligament or torn cartilage, and the X ray is negative, should the doctor get an MRI just to be sure nothing has been missed? In the face of a negative MRI, should the doctor perform exploratory arthroscopic surgery, just to be absolutely sure nothing is wrong?

Here the physical exam represents Q1 on the graph, the X ray represents Q2, the MRI is Q3, and arthroscopic surgery is Q4. The marginal benefit is measured as the increase in the probability the student's knee will be completely healed in six months. The one difference in this graph is that the cost of each successive test, rather than being constant, is increasing. How many tests should the patient obtain? In this example, the benefit derived from the physician's exam is more than the cost of the exam. The added benefit from the X ray is approximately equal to its added cost. However, the chances of an MRI helping (given a negative exam and negative X ray), though real and measurable, are less than their cost. Similarly, exploratory arthroscopic surgery not only may not help but carries with it the chance of making the patient worse from a postoperative joint infection.

Where should a rational patient stop in obtaining tests or treatments? Where should a rational physician stop in ordering these procedures? These questions are answered differently in the United States and Canada, based on our different approach to the trade-off between the benefit to the individual and the benefit of society. In Canada, technology such as MRIs is applied sparingly because it is felt that the added benefit to society overall does not justify the added cost of making it more widely available. In the United States we typically expect technology to be available to us, whatever its position on the marginal cost/marginal benefit curves. It is not fair to the individual, we believe, to deprive her of the possible benefits of the test even though they are small compared to the cost.

As in the case of consuming prime rib, the point of intersection of the marginal cost and marginal benefit curves provides a measure of efficiency in the allocation of health care resources. In Canada, tests and procedures more closely approximate Q2 on the graph, where costs and benefits are about equal. In the United States, they typically are available all the way to Q3. (Some would say we sometimes reach Q4, providing some tests and procedures that are to the patient's detriment.) Our belief in the importance of making tests and procedures available to individuals even though the marginal costs substantially exceed the marginal benefits is a uniquely American institution.

Concept 2.4

In the United States, the value we as a society place on technology and techno-logical advances encourages the development and use of high-tech medical treatments, even when the added benefit of these treatments is small compared to their cost.

The "Technological Imperative" and Its Effect on Health Care

Why is the lure of an MRI so powerful, both for the doctor and the patient? As a society we have come to put substantial faith in new technology, and often measure the benefit of a test or treatment not only by its actual ben-efit (often measured in the cost of saving an additional year of life), but also by its perceived benefit. A large part of our resistance to reducing the use of expensive, new technologies is due to what Victor Fuchs (1983, p. 60) describes as "the 'technological imperative'—namely, the desire of the physician to do everything that he has been trained to do, regardless of the benefit-cost ratio." The technological imperative shapes what we define as "best medical practice." This perception, based to a large extent on the extensive use of technology so pervasive in academic medical centers, is imprinted on physicians during their medical school and residency training. Physicians learn to do all they feasibly can, and tend to follow this institu-tional imperative throughout their career.

During much of the twentieth century, most advances in medicine were due to technological developments. New types of imaging devices such as MRI scanners, the use of fiber optics for both diagnosis and surgery, the use of lasers, and bioengineered medications all have had substantial impact on the ability to treat specific patients and specific illnesses. They have been so successful that we have come to equate technology with qual-ity. We have a commonly held belief that the more technological a treat-ment is, the better it is. We also have come to believe that as patients we have not received complete treatment unless we receive the most advanced technology. Thus physicians in the United States have a tendency to do everything that is possible, regardless of the benefit/cost ratio.

I would add to Fuchs's description a corollary institution that I call the "technological benefit of the doubt." In comparing a new, high-tech approach to a problem with an older, low-tech alternative, we tend to expect the newer approach to be superior based on its use of advanced technology, absent empirical evidence to the contrary. Take for example the prostate-specific antigen (PSA) test, which is often used as a screening device for prostate cancer. It is expensive ($50–80 per patient), and it has a high risk of false positive results. Some data suggest that widespread use of the test "may result in poorer health outcomes and will increase costs dramatically" (Krahn et al. 1994). Nonetheless, the test became widely accepted and used before it was approved by the U.S. Food and Drug Administration (FDA) and before data about its effectiveness became available. A poll found that 92% of physicians in one state used the test routinely on men over 50 (Kolata 1993). Similar data suggest that the routine use of ultrasound testing for pregnant women may offer little added benefit (Ewigman et al. 1993). Nonetheless, many patients expect ultrasound.

Physicians and patients seem willing to adopt expensive technologies on the faith that they will, in the future, prove superior to existing alternatives. Once they have been adopted, it is extremely difficult to change established patterns of behavior that prove to have little scientific or economic justification.

The Institutional Basis of Medical Malpractice

A final example of an institution with powerful effects on health care and its costs is our current malpractice system. As a society we have adopted the implicit assumption that a poor outcome from medical care implies negligence on the part of the physician. Responding to the perception that malpractice awards are based on irrational responses of lay jurors, physicians have added billions of dollars to our health care budget by ordering extra tests and procedures that add little to care but present a stronger defense in case of a malpractice suit. This practice of "defensive medicine" offers little added benefit to patients.

Negligence in medical care occurs when a doctor provides care that is not consistent with the "community standard of care"—that is, with what an expert or panel of experts would expect a reasonably competent doctor to do under similar circumstances. Thus malpractice is derived from other physicians' assessment of the quality of the care provided.

As part of a large research project, a panel of expert physicians looked at more than 30,000 hospital records in 51 different hospitals. Their independent review of these records found that hospitalized patients experienced some sort of adverse outcome from their care about 4% of the time. They then looked to see how many of the patients who experienced a bad outcome did so because the doctor or the hospital had provided substandard care (the legal basis for a finding of negligence). They found that 28% of bad outcomes could be traced to negligence (Brennan et al., 1991).

The researchers then asked, of the patients with a bad outcome who experienced substandard care, how many actually filed a malpractice lawsuit? Among the patients who received negligent care, only a tiny fraction (1–2%) actually filed a malpractice suit in response to their care.

The panel then looked at the same data in a different way. They asked, of those patients who filed malpractice suits, how many had experienced negligent care? According to this expert panel, less than 20% of the malpractice suits represented instances of negligent care. Thus when negligent care occurs, the patient usually doesn't sue, and when a patient does sue, more often than not the case doesn't actually involve negligent care. As the researchers concluded, "the civil justice system only infrequently compensates injured patients and rarely holds healthcare providers accountable for substandard care" (Localio et al. 1991, p. 250).

The panel then went on to look at the eventual judgment against the physician or hospital (if any) from the malpractice suits that were filed. They found no association between the amount of judgment received by the patient and whether the patient had received negligent care. The only factor that was associated with the level of judgment was the level of disability of the patient. The more disabled the patient as a result of treatment, the larger was the malpractice award, independent of actual negligence occurring (Brennan et al. 1996).

Another series of studies looked at a small group of obstetricians who had a record of repeated malpractice suits against them. A panel of experts compared the quality of the care provided by these doctors to the quality of care provided by comparable doctors who hadn't been sued in the past. The panel found no difference in the quality of the care between the two groups (Entman et al. 1994).

The panel again looked at the obstetricians who had been sued and those who had not. This time they evaluated patients' satisfaction with the quality of their interpersonal interaction with these doctors. The doctors who had been sued were rated much lower on this scale of quality. From the perspective of their patients, these doctors didn't communicate well, and the patients' interaction with the doctors felt more awkward (Hickson et al. 1994). It appears that the reason these obstetricians were sued and their colleagues were not was not because the quality of their care was lower; it was because they had a weaker interpersonal relationship with their patients. An editorial that accompanied this research concluded,

> The same communication skills that reduce malpractice risk lead to patient satisfaction and improved quality of care. Caring, concerned physicians who communicate well with their patients are likely to provide the best quality of care. (Levinson 1994, p. 1620)

Concept 2.5

In the United States, the institution of medical malpractice represents a combination of the following factors:

A poor outcome for the patient

A substantial level of disability as a result

A poor interpersonal relationship between the patient and the physician

Only in rare circumstances actual physician negligence

How Differing Cultural Institutions Affect the Cost of Health Care

How do differences between the United States and Canada in the organizing principles and institutions of health care affect the way care is provided and the cost of that care? We have already seen that Canada spends less than 10% of GDP on its health care system, while the United States spends nearly 14%. However, it is not simply in limiting the availability of expensive care through long waiting lists that Canada spends less than the United States. There are fundamental differences in the way physicians in the two countries practice medicine, with resulting differences in costs.

Victor Fuchs has done a number of studies comparing the patterns of care in comparable populations of patients in the United States and Canada (Fuchs 1993). The results of these comparisons have a great deal to say about why health care costs so much more in this country than it does in Canada. Table 2.2 shows the pattern of care for both physician services and hospital services. It shows the ratio of the United States to Canada in three areas: expenditures on care, prices of resources used in care, and quantity of resources used.

Several patterns can be seen from the Table 2.2. Although people in the United States go to the doctor less often (0.72 compared to Canada) and are admitted to the hospital less often (0.91), we nonetheless spend a great deal more per patient per year (1.72 for doctors' services and 1.26 for hospital care). How is it that we use care less frequently but spend a great deal more for the care? Part of the answer is the price of resources. Resources such as laboratory tests, medications, and supplies used in providing care in physicians' offices cost 30% more in the United States than comparable resources in Canada. The prices physicians charge for their services is nearly two-and-a-half times more than Canadian physicians charge. The resources used in providing hospital care also cost somewhat more in the United States (1.04).

Table 2.2   Utilization of Health Care Resources:
Ratio of United States to Canada

Physician services

Health expenditures per capita	1.72
Physicians' fees	2.39
Prices of resources used in providing service	1.30
Number of services provided per capita	0.72
Quantity of resources used per service	1.84

Hospital services

Hospital expenses per capita	1.26
Expenses per admission	1.39
Prices of resources	1.04
Hospital admissions per capita	0.91
Quantity of resources used per admission	1.24

Source: Fuchs 1993

In addition to higher prices for resources in the United States, we find a clear pattern of using more resources per service in the United States, both for physician care (1.84) and hospital care (1.24). This means that every time we go to the doctor or the hospital we get more tests, X rays, medications, and treatments than Canadians with similar conditions do. Not only do we wait less time for care, we get care involving many more resources.

Our fascination with technology, our orientation to the needs of the individual, our expectation that we will get expensive tests and procedures even if the added benefit is relatively small, and our propensity to sue doctors for malpractice all add up to care that is much more resource-intensive, and thus much more expensive. These cost differences take on even more significance when we recall that all Canadians have health insurance as a

Concept 2.6

Cultural institutions unique to the United States have helped create a health care system that is the most expensive in the world while excluding more people from care than any developed country. Any attempt to reform the system to address these problems must consider the institutions that led to the problems in the first place.

right of residency but in the United States 43 million people have no health insurance at all. Our system of care has developed in response to our dominant cultural institutions. As a consequence the U.S. system provides the most expensive care in the world while excluding the largest number of people from care.

REFERENCES

Brennan TA, Leape LL, Laird NM, et al. Incidence of Adverse Events and Negligence in Hospitalized Patients. *New England Journal of Medicine* 1991; 324:370–76.

Brennan TA, Sox CM, Burstin HR. Relation Between Negligent Adverse Events and the Outcomes of Medical-Malpractice Litigation. *New England Journal of Medicine* 1996; 335:1963–67.

DiMaggio PJ. Interest and Agency in Institutional Theory. pp. 3–21 in Zucker L. ed. *Institutional Patterns and Organizations.* Cambridge, Mass: Ballinger, 1988.

Entman SS, Glass CA, Hickson GB, et al. The Relation Between Malpractice Claims History and Subsequent Obstetrical Quality. *JAMA* 1994; 272:1588–91.

Ewigman BG, Crane JP, Frigoletto FD, et al. Effects of Prenatal Ultrasound Screening on Perinatal Outcome. *New England Journal of Medicine* 1993; 329:821–27.

Fuchs VR. *Who Shall Live.* New York: Basic Books, 1983.

Fuchs VR. The Future of Health Policy. Cambridge, MA: Harvard University Press, 1993.

Hamilton WH. *Medical Care for the American People: The Final Report of the Committee on the Cost of Medical Care, Adopted October 31, 1932.* Chicago: University of Chicago Press, 1932.

Hickson GB, Clayton EW, Entman SS, et al. Obstetricians' Prior Malpractice Experience and Patients' Satisfaction with Care. *JAMA* 1994; 272:1583–87.

Iglehart JK. Revisiting the Canadian Health Care System. *New England Journal of Medicine* 2000; 342:2007–12.

Kolata G. How Demand Surged for Unapproved Prostate Test. *New York Times.* Sept. 29, 1993. p. B7, Col. 1.

Krahn MD, Mahoney JE, Eckman MH, et al. Screening for Prostate Cancer: A Decision Analytic View. *JAMA* 1994; 272:773–80,.

Krasner SD. *International Regimes.* Ithaca, N.Y.: Cornell University Press, 1983.

Levinson W. Physician-Patient Communication, A Key to Malpractice Prevention. *JAMA* 1994, 272:1619–20.

Lipset SM. *Continental Divide.* New York: Rutledge, Chapman, and Hall, 1990.

Localio AR, Lawthers AG, Brennan TA, et al. Relation Between Malpractice Claims and Adverse Events Due to Negligence. *New England Journal of Medicine* 1991; 325: 245–51.

Meilicke CA , Storch JL, eds. *Perspectives on Canadian Health Services Policy: History and Emerging Trends.* Ann Arbor, Mich.: Health Administration Press, 1980.

North DC. Institutions, *Institutional Change and Economic Performance.* New York: Cambridge University Press, 1986.

Royal Commission on Health Services. *Report.* Ottawa: Queen's Printers, 1964.

Scott WR. The Adolescence of Institutional Theory. *Administrative Science Quarterly* 32: 493–511, 1987.

Taylor MG. *Health Insurance and Canadian Public Policy*, 2nd ed. Montreal: McGill-Queens University Press, 1987.

CHAPTER 3

The Health Professions and the Organization of Care

Key Concepts

- The American Medical Association (AMA), acting as the representative of the medical profession, was able to exert considerable power during much of the 20th century over the organization, financing, and delivery of medical care in this country.

- A primary care physician is a physician who provides continuing, comprehensive, coordinated medical care that is not differentiated by gender, disease, or organ system. Typically, primary care physicians are from one of three areas of training: family practice, general internal medicine, and general pediatrics.

- Nurse practitioners have been shown to be an effective alternative to physicians in a number of settings in terms of quality, cost, and patient satisfaction.

- A number of forces, including the higher level of income available, have encouraged the majority of young physicians to become specialists. Fewer than a third of physicians become primary care physicians.

- Historically the supply of physicians in a community has not obeyed the economic law of supply and demand. The greater the number of physicians, the greater has been the amount of care and the number of procedures. Instead of reducing the price of care, the rising number of specialist physicians has contributed to the rising cost of care.

- As a consequence of the decision by Medicare to pay for the residency training of physicians, the number of residency training positions has increased dramatically. One out of every four physicians entering residency training is a graduate of a foreign medical school. The influx of foreign medical graduates has contributed to the oversupply of specialists and thus to the rising cost of care.

- The prospective payment system coupled with the movement to outpatient surgery led to a substantial decline in hospital occupancy rates. Lower occupancy rates mean less hospital income *and* a less efficient hospital. As a result many hospitals face serious financial problems.

- There appears to be a strong direct relationship between the frequency with which a physician or facility performs a specialized medical procedure and the quality of the outcome for the patient.

The health care system in the United States is a complex combination of public and private mechanisms for providing care and paying for care. It is financed largely through health insurance, either public or private. Patients who have insurance generally pay only a small portion of the actual cost of care out of pocket, in the range of 25% of doctors' charges and 10% of hospital costs. The rest comes from insurance. Since patients rarely see the bill for their care, they usually are shielded from knowing what that care actually costs. This is in sharp contrast to other market commodities.

In addition to a wide variety of private health insurance options, there are many different types of publicly financed health insurance. These include

- Medicare, the federal program for those over 65 and the disabled
- Medicaid, the combined federal-state program for the poor
- Veterans Affairs health system, for certain categories of military veterans
- Defense Department health system, for those on active military duty
- Indian Health Service, for Native Americans both on reservations and in cities

We end up with a wide variety of payment mechanisms for health care. Each program has its own list of what is covered and what is not and how much the patient has to pay.

Regardless of what method is used for paying for care, health care decisions are still largely made by physicians. Even though physicians account for only 20% of health care expenditures, they influence between 70% and 80% of those expenditures. Medications are prescribed by physicians, tests are ordered by physicians, and patients are admitted to the hospital by physicians. Thus physicians' decisions effectively determine how much health care costs.

Physicians and the American Medical Profession

Currently we have more than 750,000 active physicians in this country, about one for every 360 people. Unfortunately they are not distributed equally. In places like Palo Alto and San Francisco, California, where it is very desirable to live and practice, there is about one physician for every 200 people. Many rural areas have one physician for every 1000 people or more. States vary widely in how many physicians they have, from one for every 230 people in Massachusetts to one per 577 people in Mississippi and Idaho (Pasko and Seidman 1999).

Doctors continue to earn one of the highest average incomes of any profession. In 1997 the median income of a physician was $164,000, with specialists earning substantially more and primary care physicians somewhat less (Zhang and Tran 1999). The median income for different specialties is shown in Figure 3.1.

Before 1900, being a doctor in the United States was not necessarily a great distinction. Although physicians were generally honored, they did not earn anywhere near the amount they do today. There were several reasons for their relative lack of occupational status. Some of the more important reasons were the following:

- *Lack of consistency in training.* Medical education was based largely on older physicians sharing the knowledge they had accumulated through experience. These physicians represented a wide range of theories of practice, many of them conflicting in the way they understood the nature of health and disease. These conflicting approaches to medical practice were referred to as "sects." The largest of the sects were the homeopaths, the osteopaths, and the allopaths. (Modern-day physicians are descended from the allopathic sect.) The quality of the education within these sects varied with the quality of the instructor, often with little scientific basis for the training offered. It wasn't until after the Flexner report in 1910 that the concept of basing medical education and practice on scientific knowledge became widely accepted. Thus one had little idea of what any particular doctor knew and whether the chances of getting better were enhanced or impaired by seeking medical care.

- *No licensure or certification, and thus no assurance of quality.* Since there was no firm scientific basis for most of medical practice there was little on which to base laws pertaining to licensure or certification. Any person with some medical training could call himself a doctor, with no body, public or private, overseeing the quality of medical practice.

- *Large numbers of doctors.* In addition to the inconsistent quality of doctors, there were large numbers of doctors. Since it was relatively easy to operate a medical school (simply provide a space for senior physicians to lecture on what they knew and find enough students who were willing to pay for obtaining that knowledge), there were large numbers of medical schools.

In the face of large numbers of doctors representing a variety of theories of illness and treatment with little in the way of scientific basis for medical practice and no assurance of quality or consistency of care, physicians were

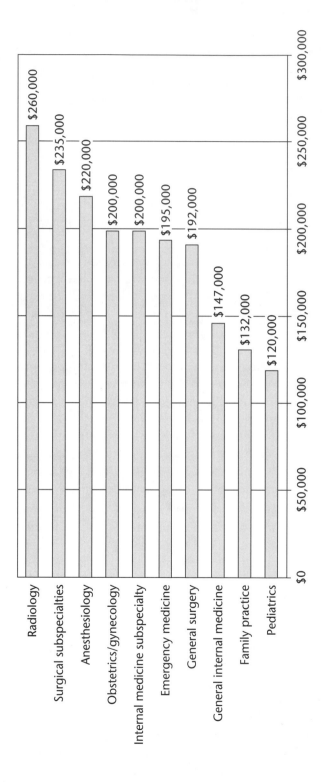

Figure 3.1 Median Income of US. Physicians in 1997, by Specialty

Source: Zhang and Tran 1999

not perceived as being in a high status profession. The income they received from medical practice was accordingly much less than what is seen today.

The American Medical Association (AMA) started out as a group of young doctors who wanted to better the doctor's lot. Most of their members were drawn from the allopathic sect of practice. For about 50 years (1846–1900), the AMA had little effect in changing the nature of medical practice.

At about this time, a new model of medical education was beginning to spread from Europe to the United States. It became established at places like Johns Hopkins and Harvard universities. Previously most medical schools were freestanding, without any association with universities. The new curriculum, supported by the Flexner report (1910), required medical schools to do the following:

1. Be part of universities

2. Have at least four years of training

3. Have the first two years of that training concentrate on basic laboratory science

Most states adopted the recommendations in the Flexner report and incorporated them into laws governing medical licensure. All new doctors, in order to be allowed to practice under these new licensure laws, had to graduate from a medical school that based its education on this model. The AMA and its state affiliates, representing allopathic physicians, were given responsibility for certifying which schools met the standard. Thus the AMA was effectively able to control the number of medical schools, and therefore the number of doctors, in the United States, and to establish the criteria for licensure.

The overall quality and consistency of medical training and practice improved substantially—as did the income of doctors, due largely to their shrinking numbers. In addition the new medical schools provided a place for medical research. Most medical advances in the twentieth century were developed in medical schools.

The AMA also worked to establish control over the manufacture of pharmaceuticals. Only the companies that pledged to follow the AMA's code of ethics were approved and allowed to advertise in the AMA's journals (Starr 1982). Doctors were discouraged from prescribing drugs that did not have the AMA's approval. As a result, a mutually dependent relationship developed between the drug companies and the AMA, and the drug companies came to be very powerful. They formed their own association, the Pharmaceutical Research and Manufacturers of America (PRMA) (formerly the Pharmaceutical Manufacturers' Association, or PMA). Over the years the power of the PRMA, both scientifically and politically, paralleled that of the AMA. Through its support of laws providing patent protection for new drugs and extensive marketing of new (often extremely expensive) drugs, the pharmaceutical industry has been able to maintain one of the highest profit margins of any American industry. Through their extensive program of medical research, pharmaceutical companies have provided many important advances in treatment, but they have also provided many expensive new drugs that offer relatively little benefit over older, less expensive drugs. As a result, the cost of drugs has been a major contributor to the rising cost of health care.

Building on its grant of authority over medical school certification and medical licensure, the AMA also came to define the code of ethics that physicians must follow (Baker et al. 1999). This code of ethics covered not only issues of medical practice but also issues of medical economics. From rules governing the physician-patient relationship to methods of organizing and paying for medical practice, the AMA gained nearly total authority over physicians. This code of ethics was applied not just to physicians who were members of the AMA, but to all physicians. As we see in Chapter 4 as part of our consideration of the origin of health maintenance organizations, this extension of ethical standards to include the organization of medical practice led to significant splits within the profession. These splits were to have important ramifications for the efforts at health care reform we have seen in this country over the last 20 years.

Today the AMA represents fewer than half of all physicians, but is still the most powerful voice of the medical profession on matters of medical ethics, medical education, and the standards of medical practice. In addition, the AMA has for years been one of the biggest contributors to politicians, and has one of the most powerful lobbying organizations in Washington, D.C. During much of the twentieth century the power of the AMA was such that it was repeatedly able to block efforts in Congress to establish a system of universal health coverage.

Concept 3.1

The American Medical Association (AMA), acting as the representative of the medical profession, was able to exert considerable power during much of the twentieth century over the organization, financing, and delivery of medical care in this country.

Racial Segregation and the Medical Profession

For much of its history, the AMA excluded African-American physicians from membership. In addition, African-American physicians were frequently blocked at the local level from joining the medical staff of predominantly white hospitals. Thus as part of the history of racial segregation in this country we maintained a segregated system of medical education and medical care, based to a large extent on the policies promulgated by the AMA (Smith 1999).

In the period following the Civil War a small number of predominantly black medical schools gained substantial respect. Foremost among these were Howard University and Meharry Medical College. In the 1890s the graduates of these schools, prevented from joining the AMA, formed a separate association—the National Medical Association (NMA)—to represent African-American physicians. In the 1950s the AMA and its affiliated state medical associations began to extend membership to African-American physicians, although it wasn't until the 1960s following enactment of the Civil Rights Act that African-American physicians became full members of the American medical profession.

Until the 1960s there existed in many parts of this country a system of overt segregation of white and nonwhite hospitals. Black physicians were not allowed on the medical staff of many white hospitals and black patients were not allowed treatment. Congress then passed both landmark civil rights legislation and the laws creating the Medicare and Medicaid programs. Together these programs extended the availability of hospital care to the poor and the elderly and as a result became a major source of funding for most hospitals. Those responsible for enacting Medicare and Medicaid made it clear that any hospital that continued a policy of racial segregation would be in violation of the Civil Rights Act and would be ineligible for payment under either program. Few hospitals could continue to survive without any federal funding. As a result there was a rapid dismantling of the segregated hospital system.

The NMA continues to exist as an independent association of physicians, and continues to be active in efforts to increase the number of medical students and physicians from underrepresented ethnic minorities. The relatively low numbers of African Americans and other ethnic minorities in the American medical profession continues to be a problem. For example, although African Americans currently compose about 13% of the overall United States population, only about 4% of physicians in the United States are African American. Coincident with the decreasing emphasis on affirmative action programs at many universities, the number of medical students from underrepresented ethnic minorities fell 15% between 1994 and 2000 (Schemo 2000).

Gender Segregation and the Medical Profession

For much of the early part of the twentieth century women were not allowed membership in the AMA. This reflected a generally held view that women were inappropriate as physicians. A number of medical schools refused to admit women as students, and those that did admitted only a small number. Many of the women physicians in this country were educated in women-only medical schools. Following the success of the women's suffrage movement in the 1920s, the AMA and the rest of the medical profession began to open its ranks to women.

When, as a medical student in the 1970s, this author served as a member of the admissions committee of a nationally prestigious medical school, women applicants were given extra scrutiny to ensure that their interest in establishing a family did not conflict with their interest in becoming a physician. As a result fewer than 10 percent of medical students at that school and nationwide were women. As women in this country have attained increasing status relative to men, their numbers in the medical profession have increased accordingly. Today nearly half of all medical students (more than half at some schools) are women. Over time medicine will become a profession with as many women physicians as men.

Nursing in the United States

Another important profession in United States health care is nursing. Interestingly, the history of the nursing profession is also the history of war. Nursing was formed as a profession in the 1800s through the efforts of Florence Nightingale and others on the battlefields of the Crimean War. Following a growing public awareness of her work, schools of nursing began to be established in the United Kingdom and the United States.

Due to a shortage of nurses in World War I, a new category of subnurse was created, which eventually became the medical assistant. Today medical assistants frequently work under the direction of registered nurses in both hospital and medical office settings. Another shortage of nursing personnel during World War II led to the creation of a third category of nurse, the licensed vocational nurse, or LVN. Today hospitals, clinics, and doctors' offices employ a combination of medical assistants, LVNs, and registered nurses, or RNs.

At the same time that the university-based medical school was spreading to this country, the model of the hospital-based nursing school was also spreading. Previously, nursing education had been as varied and haphazard as medical education. In 1911 a group of alumnae from these hospital-based schools formed an association and argued that only graduates of these schools should be licensed to act as nurses. This was the birth of the American Nursing Association, or ANA. The ANA has never been as powerful as the AMA. To a large extent, it has acted in the role of a collective bargaining agent in nurses' struggle with hospitals to gain the professional status and level of pay that the profession deserved. In this effort, there were often rival labor unions for nurses, with a result that the profession had difficulty becoming unified.

More recently, the ANA has been involved in discussions of further upgrading the level of training and skills required of nursing graduates. The traditional hospital-based training programs were two years long. Many nurses argue that all nurses should have four years of education, the equivalent of a college education. Those nurses who complete a full four years of education receive a baccalaureate degree and are referred to as baccalaureate nurses. Over time the baccalaureate has come to replace the certificate nurse (i.e., a nurse graduating from a shorter hospital-based training program) in most medical settings.

Many nurses have been able to upgrade their training through specialized programs to form highly skilled subgroups within the profession. For example, emergency room nurses, coronary care nurses, and neonatal care nurses have become indispensable members of the critical care teams in hospitals and have considerable autonomy in the care of patients. In addition, several types of nurses have been able to obtain extra training to act as semi-independent practitioners, discussed below.

Primary Care and the Role of Primary Care Physicians

In examining health care in the United States it is possible to divide our system into multiple levels:

- Primary care: care provided by doctors' offices and clinics
- Secondary care: care obtained from specialists and in hospitals
- Tertiary care: care obtained at regional referral centers
- Quaternary care: care obtained at national referral centers

We look at each of these levels separately in the remainder of the chapter.

There has been a great deal of discussion among physicians, among patients, and in the media about the role of primary care physicians. In these discussions it is important to be specific in defining "primary care." There are at least two ways of approaching primary care and defining which physicians are primary care physicians.

1. *The disease-oriented approach:* physicians who provide the first stage of treatment for a disease

By this definition of primary care nearly any type of doctor can be considered a primary care physician, depending on the nature of the illness. The following examples illustrate this approach to primary care:

- You see your family doctor for treatment of a sore throat
- You consult a dermatologist for treatment of acne
- You seek prenatal care from an obstetrician
- You consult a cardiologist regarding chest pains you experience
- You are treated by an emergency physician for injuries sustained in an auto accident.

2. *The person-oriented approach:* a physician who provides continuing, comprehensive, coordinated medical care that is not differentiated by gender, disease, or organ system

Under this definition only those physicians who treat a comprehensive range of problems, getting to know a patient and his health status over time, are considered primary care physicians. From this approach only physicians with training in one of three specialties are considered to be primary care physicians: family practice, general internal medicine, and general pediatrics.

An obstetrician would not be considered a primary care physician because her practice is gender-specific. A cardiologist or dermatologist would not be a primary care physician because each practice is limited to one organ system. An emergency physician, although treating a comprehensive range of problems, would not be a primary care physician because he does not develop a continuous relationship with a patient over time.

Concept 3.2

A primary care physician is a physician who provides continuing, comprehensive, coordinated medical care that is not differentiated by gender, disease, or organ system. Typically, primary care physicians are from one of three areas of training: family practice, general internal medicine, and general pediatrics.

The recent debate over health care reform has focused a great deal of attention on the need for primary care physicians. For a period in the 1990s it appeared that there was a crisis due to the falling number of primary care physicians. Lured by the prestige of being a specialist, fewer and fewer medical students were choosing a career in primary care. In 1982 about one-third of all medical students indicated that they planned to enter primary care. In 1992 fewer than 20 percent of medical students opted for primary care. In recent years there has been a turnaround in this area, with a third of graduating medical students now entering primary care residencies. It remains to be seen how many of these will stay in primary care and how many will eventually subspecialize.

The perceived crisis in primary care was due partly to the increasing role of primary care physicians and partly to the realization that relatively few young doctors have been choosing to enter primary care. Reasons medical students choose to be specialists rather than primary care physicians include the following:

- *Prestige*. Specialists tend to deal with new technology; primary care physicians deal mainly with people. With our emphasis on technology as the basis of medical advances, physicians who use technology in their practice are frequently granted higher prestige, both by the profession and by society.

- *Money*. As indicated in Figure 3.1 previously, some specialists earn more than twice as much as primary care physicians. Following large cutbacks in the 1980s in financial aid for medical students, many students have had to rely on student loans to pay for their education. A number of students come out of medical school owing more than $100,000. Many feel they need the higher salary available to specialists to pay off their loans.

- *Frustration of primary care*. Primary care is often viewed by medical students as boring and repetitive, dealing mostly with common problems and chronic illnesses for which there is no cure. Specialists tend to deal with exciting, interesting problems, and to offer the hope of a cure for patients' problems.

- *Lack of primary care role models*. Most physicians who teach in medical schools are specialists. Medical students come in contact with few practicing primary care physicians. Students are often counseled by their teachers to stay away from primary care—not to "waste" their career.

However. there are also reasons primary care is an attractive career option for many students, and may be getting more attention from medical students than it did just a few years ago.

- *Employability*. One factor that may be working in the favor of primary care physicians is their ability to find employment after their training. A recent study showed that for doctors just completing their residencies, relatively few primary care doctors had difficulty in finding employment, while as many as half of all doctors in certain subspecialties reported trouble finding employment (Miller et al. 1998). One reason for this advantage in employment has been the increasing role of primary care physicians in health maintenance organizations and other types of managed care settings. (We discuss the origins of managed care systems in Chapter 4.) In traditional medical practice, a number of specialists did not have enough patients to fill their practice, so they would spend part of their time giving specialized care and part of their time giving primary care. In the managed care setting most specialists provide only specialty care, with the result that fewer specialists and more primary care physicians are needed in these practice settings.

■ *The nontangible benefits of primary care practice.* It may be true that primary care physicians frequently deal with common problems and chronic illness, but there is an aspect to this type of medical practice that many medical students are not aware of. In getting to know patients and their families over time and in dealing with the problems that most commonly confront patients, primary care physicians are able to develop a unique type of relationship with their patients. Patients tend to trust and admire the physician who is there for them day in and day out. It is difficult to put a dollar value on the strength of the interpersonal relationship many primary physicians are able to establish with their patients. This can be the most rewarding aspect of primary care practice. Physicians who value the quality of their relationship with their patients over professional prestige and income are frequently at home in primary care practice, and usually make the best primary care physicians.

Currently about 30% of physicians in the United States are in primary care. Many people argue that we need to increase this number to about 50% of doctors, as in Canada. Others respond that if we had 50% of physicians in primary care there would be a shortage of specialists. Recall that Canada provides a great deal less specialized care than we do, and thus needs fewer specialists. It may be that we couldn't keep up our current level of specialized care with only 50% of doctors as specialists. Policies adopted to influence the number of primary care physicians (and thus the number of specialists) will thus play an important role in determining the direction our health care system will take.

It is true that, as a percentage of the medical profession, primary care has fallen steadily over time. However, as illustrated in Figure 3.2, the number of primary care physicians per 100,000 people has changed little over the last 50 years.

In the period 1950–1960, when nearly two-thirds of physicians were in primary care, there were about 90 primary care physicians for every 100,000 people in the country. In the period 1990-2000, when primary care physicians were less than one-third of all physicians, there were about 80 primary care physicians per 100,000 population. Since 1950 we have had about the same number of primary care physicians per 100,000 popu-

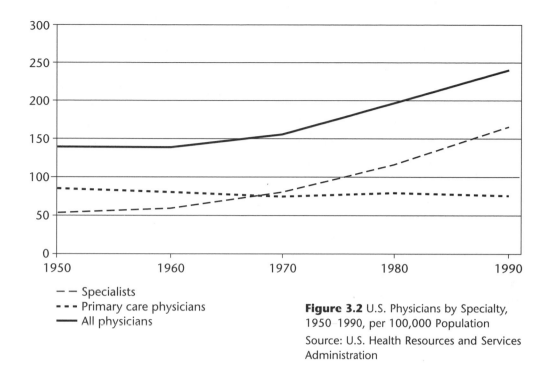

Figure 3.2 U.S. Physicians by Specialty, 1950 1990, per 100,000 Population

Source: U.S. Health Resources and Services Administration

— — Specialists
- - - Primary care physicians
—— All physicians

lation. During this time there has been a 75 percent increase in the total number of physicians per 100,000 population. Almost all of the increase has been specialists. In actuality we have about the same number of primary care physicians we have always had when measured this way. The increasing number of specialists has led to the declining percentage of physicians who are in primary care. The problems may not be a shortage of primary care physicians; it may be an excess of specialists.

Nurse Practitioners and Other Advanced Practice Nurses

An alternative to training primary care physicians is training advanced practice nurses. Most common are the nurse practitioner (NP) and nurse midwife. NPs take two to three years of training beyond the RN level, part of it a clinical internship. They can be trained in family medicine, adult medicine, pediatrics, or obstetrics. Following their training, NPs are eligible to see and treat patients for specified conditions under the supervision of a physician. The physician does not have to be present to provide supervision. The physician and the NP don't even have to be in the same office. NPs typically work from written treatment protocols worked out with their physician, and refer all things beyond their capabilities to the supervising physician. (Physician assistants differ from NPs in not being nurses, in having to work more directly under the supervision of a physician, and in being more limited in what they can do.)

There was a movement to train more NPs in the 1970s due to the perception of a nationwide physician shortage. With the recent perceptions of a shortage of primary care physicians, there is again a movement to train NPs. There currently are about 50,000 NPs.

A problem has been that many physicians are not comfortable either supervising NPs or having their patients seen by NPs. However, repeated studies have shown that NPs can give care that is the same quality as physicians for the specific conditions they are trained for. The studies also show that patients accept NPs quite well. In many cases patients are more satisfied with care by an NP than by a physician, due largely to the extra time and personal attention NPs are able to give. NPs seem especially well suited for medical conditions in which a great deal of face-to-face contact is required, such as well child care, arthritis, diabetes, and high blood pressure (United States Office of Technology Assessment 1986; Salkever et al. 1982; Maule 1994).

The question remains unanswered as to whether care provided by NPs costs less than care provided by physicians. Because they spend more time with patients, they see fewer patients. A study done in the 1980s by the Kaiser-Permanente system of care in northern California found that overall care from nurse practitioners cost about the same as physician care, but patients liked them better than doctors in the clinic (Garfield et al. 1987).

Concept 3.3

Nurse practitioners have been shown to be an effective alternative to physicians in a number of settings in terms of quality, cost, and patient satisfaction.

Perhaps a more important issue than whether to train more primary care physicians or nurse practitioners is how primary care should be organized as part of managed care. With the spread of managed care plans, primary care is increasingly being provided by large groups of physicians. The solo doctor, practicing alone in his or her own office, has largely become a thing of the past. Many people suggest that we need to look at new ways of organizing primary care practice so as to maintain the quality of the primary care process and make it readily accessible to patients.

One possible solution would be community-oriented primary care (COPC) (Wright 1993). COPC takes an ecological approach to health care, seeing illness and injury as affected by environmental and social factors.

The best way to approach health care under this perspective is to base primary care practice in the community rather than in large, centralized clinic facilities. An interdisciplinary health care team then provides primary care for an identifiable population of patients. Part of the care is monitoring conditions in the community. This model differs from the traditional and still predominant model in which physicians have little actual contact with or awareness of the community in which the patients live. Much research needs to be done to identify the best ways to provide primary care, particularly as part of large, managed care organizations. Perhaps models that have both physicians and nurse practitioners working in close collaboration as part of a health care team provides a promising solution to the need for more primary care practitioners.

Secondary Care—Specialist Physicians

As discussed earlier, physicians are separated into two categories: primary care physicians and specialists. Specialists are those physicians who have received extra training in a specific field, and who treat only a certain type of patient. The point at which primary care physicians and specialists become identified and differentiated is during residency training. Nearly every medical student goes on after medical school to receive additional training in a residency. Residencies are usually based in a hospital and have faculty drawn from a specific field of medicine.

The concept of the "internship" no longer applies to medical training in the United States. During much of the twentieth century, medical students would initially complete a one-year, hospital-based training after medical school (the internship), and then go on to a separate residency training program. Over time it has become the standard that the first year of training after medical school is part of residency training, often referred to as the R1 year. It is possible to obtain a license to practice medicine in many states after the R1 year, but fewer and fewer students stop at this level of training. In the past, those physicians who stopped after one year of extra training were referred to as general practitioners, or GPs. GPs have largely been replaced by family practitioners and other types of primary care physicians with a full three years of residency training.

The length of residency training can vary significantly, depending on the area of specialty. Emergency room specialists complete their residency training in three years; certain types of surgeons (e.g., cardiac surgeons or neurosurgeons) can take eight or more years before completing training. Some areas of specialty may require two separate residencies, such as an initial period of residency in general surgery followed by a separate residency in orthopedic surgery.

A number of specialists in nonsurgical fields may start out their train-ing in the same program as primary care physicians, but then go on to take extra training in a specialized field within their discipline. For example, stu-dents wishing to become cardiologists (heart specialists) or gastroenterolo-gists (intestinal specialists) will often take the same three-year residency in general internal medicine as primary care physicians, but go on to take a "fellowship" in their specialized area of interest. Similarly, a physician com-pleting a residency in general pediatrics may go on to a fellowship in neona-tology (the care of premature babies and other newborns). A fellowship is distinguished from a residency in that it is available only to those who have completed more general training in a specific field, and it provides training in only one segment of that field. Fellowships are typically between two and four years long.

As indicated in Figure 3.1 shown previously, most specialists have an income that is considerably higher than that of primary care physicians. By spending a few extra years in training, physicians can nearly double their expected earning power. Although this differential in income between spe-cialists and primary care physicians has recently declined somewhat, the higher income a specialist can expect to earn continues to play a major role in drawing students into these areas. In addition, many young physicians want to use the latest technology in their practice, or to have the challenge of performing surgery with its attendant risks for the patient. The majority of medical students continue to choose careers in medical specialties.

Concept 3.4

A number of forces, including the higher level of income available, have encour-aged the majority of young physicians to become specialists. Fewer than a third of physicians become primary care physicians.

Since the changes in medical practice that accompanied the shift to man-aged care in this country, the way a specialist practices medicine has changed substantially. Previously, any patient who wanted to consult a specialist about a problem simply called the specialist's office and made an appointment. Because specialty care tends to be more expensive than primary care, many insurance companies and managed care companies have placed limits on patients' ability to be seen by the specialist of their choice. Now many patients must first seek care from their primary care physician, and will have the care of a specialist covered under their medical insurance only if it is first approved by the primary care physician. In addition, certain types of specialists use expensive tests and procedures as part of their practice. In an effort to control costs, many insurance companies require these specialists to obtain permission from the insurance company before providing expensive care. These two limitations on the practice of specialists—"gatekeepers" and "prior authorization"—are discussed in more depth in Chapter 4.

The rising number of specialists, both in absolute numbers and as a percentage of the medical profession, raises serious concerns about the contribution of this situation to the rising cost of care. As in many areas of medical care, changes in the number of specialist physicians do not necessarily lead to changes in the price of specialty care. If your community had a sudden increase in the number of house painters working, you could reasonably expect the cost of having your house painted to go down. With most market commodities, as the supply of a commodity (such as house painters) goes up, the price should come down. Despite the market approach to medical care prevalent in this country for most of the twentieth century, the market for physicians did not seem to obey the laws of supply and demand. Instead, physicians were able to avoid becoming a surplus commodity by increasing the amount of care they provide. In the case of medical care the demand for the commodity (i.e., medical care) is determined not by the consumer but by the provider. Patients don't typically tell physicians how much and what type of care they need; physicians tell patients. Medical care in this case becomes a "market failure," in that it does not obey the classical laws of the market economy such as supply and demand (Arrow 1963).

A fundamental reality of twentieth century American medical care has been demonstrated again and again: the more specialists practicing in a given community, the more specialty care will be recommended to patients, and the higher the total cost of care. If more surgeons move into a community (all else being equal), there will be more operations. For a variety of medical conditions and geographic locations, John Wennberg and his colleagues have demonstrated a tremendous variation among communities in the rate at which certain types of specialized therapy are applied. Whether it is rates of prostate surgery or rates of heart surgery, Wennberg has concluded that a major factor

---

Concept 3.5

Historically the supply of physicians in a community has not obeyed the economic law of supply and demand. The greater the number of physicians, the greater has been the amount of care and the number of procedures. Instead of reducing the price of care, the rising number of specialist physicians has contributed to the rising cost of care.

driving the different rates of these procedures is the number of doctors practicing in the community: the more doctors, the higher the rate of surgery (Wennberg and Gittelsohn 1973, Wennberg et al, 1982, Wennberg 1993).

Foreign Medical Graduates and Their Effect on the Medical Profession

Two policy decisions have combined to encourage young physicians completing medical school in other countries to come to the United States to live and practice medicine. The first decision was to create flexibility in immigration laws to allow hospitals in the United States that are unable to fill all their residency training slots with graduates of United States medical schools to fill those slots with graduates of foreign medical schools. These foreign medical graduates, or FMGs, must first pass two standardized examinations: one documenting that they have received a medical education equivalent to that in the United States, and one documenting facility in written and spoken English. Those FMGs who successfully complete these exams are allowed to apply to United States hospitals for residency training. FMGs who obtain a residency training slot are then eligible to receive a visa to enter the United States for the duration of the residency. The intent of this immigration law is that the doctor will return to the country of origin after completion of training. However, in recent years a substantial majority of FMGs completing their training have been able to obtain permanent resident status and remain in this country.

The second policy that facilitated the employment of FMGs by hospitals in the United States was the decision by the federal Medicare program to reimburse hospitals for the cost of residency training, without limits on either numbers or types of residencies. The history of this policy is an unusual one. A relatively minor policy decision in the 1960s, unrelated to the issue of FMGs, has had the unintended long-term consequence of encouraging the immigration of large numbers of physicians.

When the Medicare program was first approved by Congress in the 1960s, the federal government used a complex formula to calculate how much to pay hospitals for treating Medicare patients. The formula allowed the hospital to obtain reimbursement for a share of the costs of running the hospital. A somewhat lengthy list was established detailing which expenses the hospital could include in calculating the federal government's share. One item included on this list was the cost of any residency training programs the hospitals might have. When Medicare switched to its prospective payment system for reimbursing hospitals (discussed below), hospitals that previously had included the costs of residency training in their payment formula were allowed to continue to bill Medicare for these costs *in addition* to the prospective payment. This policy was originally intended to allow hospitals with existing residency training programs to continue their previous level of reimbursement, but it soon became apparent that newly established residency programs were also eligible for federal reimbursement. Unintentionally, the Medicare program had written a blank check to hospitals to expand residency teaching programs. Hospitals were quick to respond. Adding a residency program (or expanding an existing one) not only adds to the prestige of the hospital, it also provides a source of inexpensive labor. In many hospitals, especially inner-city hospitals providing care to a large number of poor patients, residents provide the bulk of direct patient care.

As a result of the expansion in residency training programs, paid for by the federal government, the number of entry-level training slots has become substantially larger than the number of medical students graduating each year from United States medical schools (referred to as USMGs). USMGs tend not to choose many of the inner-city hospitals for their training, leaving large numbers of unfilled training slots at these hospitals. In order to have sufficient manpower to take care of patients, these hospitals turn to FMGs to fill the residency programs. Hospitals in cities such as New York, Chicago, and Los Angeles that once had no problem filling their residencies with USMGs now train mostly FMGs. In 1999 there were 15,566 USMGs and 5134 FMGs entering residency training in the United States (Miller et al. 1999).

The expansion of training that followed the federal government's decision to subsidize residency training has resulted in increasingly rapid growth in the number of physicians in the United States. In addition, since FMGs are more likely than USMGs to become specialists rather than primary care physicians, the policy has been a major factor contributing to the growing number of specialists in the country. The government's response to this problem is discussed in the section following on policy directions.

Concept 3.6

As a consequence of the decision by Medicare to pay for the residency training of physicians, the number of residency training positions has increased dramatically. One out of every four physicians entering residency training is a graduate of a foreign medical school. The influx of FMGs has contributed to the oversupply of specialists and thus to the rising cost of care.

Future Policy Directions for Physician Supply and Specialty

The preceding data raise the question of whether we should establish explicit policies to alter the supply of physicians in this country. The two principal options under discussion have been decreasing the number of new physicians and encouraging more young physicians to enter primary care.

Decreasing the Number of Physicians

In the 1970s there was a considerable expansion in both the number of medical schools in this country and the number of medical students in each school. These changes were in large part a response to new federal policies that provided considerable financial incentive to increase the supply of physicians. At that time there was a widely held perception that our country was facing a serious shortage of physicians. Now that we appear to have too many physicians, there has been a substantial decrease in federal funding for medical schools and medical students. In addition, many state governments are looking seriously at either shrinking the enrollment at state-supported schools or perhaps even closing some medical schools altogether. In the last several years the number of medical students in this country has remained relatively stable, although the number of applicants has dropped substantially (Association of American Medical Colleges 2000). A reduction in the number of students may necessitate even more stringent reductions in public funding for medical education.

A more focused effort is beginning to take shape to reduce the number of physicians (or at least slow the increase in the number of physicians) by attempting to reduce the number of FMGs entering this country. In a program initiated in New York, the federal government has negotiated a reduction in the number of residency training slots at a number of hospitals that historically have relied on FMGs. Under this plan, hospitals that agree to decrease the number of residency positions they offer continue to receive the federal subsidy for the positions they drop. The subsidy is phased out over a period of several years. In this way the hospital is not faced with a sudden decrease in funding, and can take the phase-out period to identify other means to provide the patient care that previously had been provided by the trainees in the residency program. This program is being expanded to hospitals in other areas of the country. Studies are under way to evaluate the success of the program in reducing the number of FMGs entering this country and the effect of the program on patient care at participating hospitals.

Increasing the Number of Primary Care Physicians

Policy makers at the federal and state level are also looking at ways to increase the number of young physicians going into primary care. Four principal options are available to accomplish this goal.

1. *Mandate that medical schools train more primary care physicians.* This option is possible mostly at state-funded universities. A number of state legislatures, responding to the public perception of a need for more primary care physicians in the state, have linked state funding to the medical school's success in training primary care physicians. In addition a number of state universities have initiated new programs to give students experience in rural primary care in an effort to increase the number of primary care physicians in these areas.

2. *Provide financial incentives for medical students to choose a career in primary care.* The federal government currently has a program to assist young physicians in repaying their student loans if they spend a period of time in a rural primary care setting after completing their training. This type of loan repayment could be expanded to include all physicians who enter primary care. In addition, medical school loans could be made preferentially available to students committing to a primary care career.

3. *Increase the emphasis on primary care in medical school and residency training.* A number of medical schools are seeking to encourage students to enter primary care by providing more role models for primary care in medical school. Sociological studies have shown how medical students can be powerfully affected in their career choices by the faculty they encounter in medical school. Expanding and strengthening the number of primary care faculty in medical schools would give more students a positive exposure to primary care, and could be expected to encourage more of them to choose a primary care career. In addition, federal funding for residency training, already being reduced, could be allocated preferentially to primary care training programs, with reductions in funding selectively affecting programs that train specialists.

4. *Allow the private market for medical care to determine the number of primary care physicians.* As mentioned above, the growing number of physicians coupled with the disproportionate number who choose to specialize has begun to affect the job prospects of recent medical graduates. In a number of medical specialties, job prospects are especially dim and average incomes have fallen substantially. In contrast, the income of primary care physicians has remained relatively stable, and the job prospects for young primary care physicians remain attractive. Many analysts attribute the recent increase in the number of medical students expressing an interest in primary care to these market forces,

and argue that the private market for medical care will be effective in determining the appropriate mix of specialists and primary care physicians for this country.

Also, the federal government's Medicare program has made a number of changes in the way it pays physicians, with the result that the income differential between primary care physicians and specialists has been reduced. The resource-based relative value scale and other policy changes in federal payment to physicians are discussed in Chapter 5.

Secondary Care—The Hospital

Throughout much of history hospitals were not places of healing—they were places to die, mostly for poor people. It was during the Napoleonic wars that doctors first started treating all of the wounded and sick soldiers in one place. Hospitals gradually became a place for the scientific study of medicine instead of a place for poor people to go to die. As part of the shift to medicine as a science-based discipline in the early twentieth century, hospitals increasingly became important for treating ill patients in an effort to prevent death. Following the Flexner report on medical education and the affiliation of medical schools with universities, hospitals became the principal location for medical research, especially university-based hospitals. Thus the hospital as we know it is a relatively young institution.

During the depression of the 1930s, patients often could not pay their hospital bill, with the result that many hospitals had a hard time staying open. Hospitals decided to group together to offer, for the first time, insurance to cover the cost of hospital care. The hope was that people who could not afford to pay a large hospital bill once they got sick could afford monthly insurance premiums to protect themselves from a large hospital bill in case they got sick. These hospital-sponsored insurance plans were the origin of the nationwide Blue Cross program. Every state had its own program of Blue Cross hospital insurance. Some states added an option for insuring against the cost of physicians' services. These were the Blue Shield plans. The AMA and its local affiliates supported the establishment of the Blue Cross/Blue Shield program so long as doctors maintained control over all medical decisions within the hospital.

In much of Europe, specialist physicians typically work only in the hospital, with primary care physicians working only in the community. When a community physician has a patient that needs to be hospitalized, the patient is often referred to the hospital-based specialist. In the United States, community physicians admit their patients to the hospital and supervise their care while they are in the hospital. This arrangement gives community physicians in the United States substantially more authority over hospital policies and practices than their counterparts in Europe.

Hospitals in the United States generally have a dual system of administration. The physicians who treat patients in the hospital are members of the medical staff. No physician may treat a patient in the hospital unless he has first been accepted for membership on the medical staff. The medical staff governs all aspects of hospital care relating to physician care, such as quality review. A nonphysician hospital administrator governs all other nonphysician aspects of hospital activities, such as the nursing, managerial/administrative, and facilities staffs. Most hospitals have an executive committee where the leaders of the medical staff and hospital administrators can jointly discuss hospital management issues.

Hospitals in the United States are more expensive both per day and per stay than in European countries and Canada. Part of the reason for this is that up until 1983 hospitals had no incentives to limit the amount of care they offered. In fact, the payment system encouraged the acquisition of new facilities and technology, even if they duplicated facilities and services readily available elsewhere in the community.

Since the 1940s a government program (the Hill-Burton program) financed the construction of new hospitals throughout the country, many of them in rural communities. In addition, the federal Medicare program (see Chapter 5) included a payment formula that reimbursed hospitals for a large part of the cost of new technology. The result was considerable expansion of the number of hospital beds and the level of hospital technology throughout the country. For most patients, hospitals simply submitted bills to insurance companies (or the federal government, in the case of Medicare) and were fully reimbursed. There was little questioning of whether the care or the cost of care was appropriate.

Since the federal government pays about 40% of hospital bills throughout the country, primarily through the Medicare and Medicaid programs, it was beginning to cost the federal government a huge amount to continue simply to reimburse hospitals for whatever they spent taking care of patients. The federal government came up with a series of plans to reduce that cost. The first, in the 1970s, was the system of professional standards review organizations, or PSROs. PSROs were groups of local physicians who would review the care provided to Medicare and Medicaid patients to ensure that it was appropriate. Although this effort was well intentioned, it had very little effect, and hospital costs continued to rise.

In an effort to reduce rapidly rising costs, the federal government established a new program. Under this program, rather than simply reimbursing a hospital for the costs of care after the fact, the Medicare program began to pay a fixed amount each time a patient was admitted to the hospital. This plan has two names: the diagnosis-related groups system (DRG), and the prospective payment system (PPS). Both names mean the same thing. Under PPS, instead of paying the hospital for each individual service, the government pays hospitals a fixed amount based on how much, on average, it should cost to take care of a patient of this type. (The PPS system currently covers only hospital costs. Physicians' charges are paid under a completely different system.) The amount of payment is based on what is wrong with the patient. For example, if a patient comes to the hospital with a heart attack that has no complications, the government has calculated how much it costs on average to take care of such a patient. This is how much the hospital gets paid, regardless of what the hospital does to treat the patient. If the patient has a heart attack with complications, the payment is more, based on the average of what it takes to take care of such a patient. The same goes for treating pneumonia, appendicitis, or breast cancer. For each type of illness, or diagnosis-related group, the government pays a fixed amount. If the hospital is able to provide care for the patient for a lower cost than what the government pays, then the hospital gets to keep the difference. If the hospital's care costs more than the government pays, then the hospital has to absorb the difference.

Under the previous payment system, with few controls on what the hospital could charge, the incentive was to keep the patient in the hospital as long as possible. Clearly the incentive under the PPS system is to get patients out of the hospital as quickly as possible. This led to many hospitals sending many patients home (or to less expensive nursing homes) before they were fully recovered. The claim was made that hospitals were discharging patients "quicker and sicker." In order to counteract this tendency and also to ensure that patients admitted to the hospital had a legitimate need for hospital care, the federal government replaced the PSRO system with one of peer review organizations, or PROs. A PRO is a local corporation that contracts with the government to provide oversight of the quality and necessity of the hospital care provided to Medicare patients. Although many PROs have considerable participation by local medical associations, they give physicians substantially less control over the review of hospital care than under the previous PSRO system.

What the prospective payment system has done is completely reverse the financial incentives faced by hospitals that provide care to Medicare patients. The result was that between 1983 and 1993, there was a substantial decrease in the average length of hospital stay. Since patients were staying in the hospital fewer days, it meant that fewer hospitals beds had patients in them at any one time. Fewer patients in the hospital means less money for the hospital. The reduction in hospital use following initiation of the PPS system resulted in substantially decreased revenues for hospitals.

An additional factor has also placed a financial squeeze on hospitals. Both the federal PPS program and many private health insurers began to encourage outpatient treatment of many conditions that formerly were treated in the hospital. In 1981 only about one out of six of operations were performed on an outpatient basis, with the rest performed in the hospital. In 1991 about half of all operations were performed on an outpatient basis. Operations such as gallbladder surgery and knee surgery that previously had kept the patient in the hospital for several days were now being done in outpatient "surgi-centers," with the patient going home the same day. Many patients now being treated as outpatients used to be treated in hospitals. Again, the result was that hospital revenues went down substantially.

The net result of these changes has been a decrease in the number of patients in the hospital on any given day, that is, a decrease in the hospital occupancy rate. Currently, a typical hospital may have 50% of its beds empty on any given day. This presents a serious problem because of the following relationships.

Hospital expenses break down according to the following proportions (Iglehart 1993):

- Labor costs: 54%
- Nonlabor costs: 37%
- Capital: 9%

Of the labor and nonlabor costs, some are fixed and some are variable. An example of fixed costs is the need for a hospital administrator. You have to have a hospital administrator no matter how many patients are in the hospital. An example of variable costs is the number of nurses working on any given day. It is possible to adjust the number of nurses working based on the number of patients in the hospital. If a hospital is only 1% full, almost all the costs are fixed costs. If a hospital is 100% full, most of the costs are variable costs. The lower the occupancy rate, the fewer patients there are to share the fixed costs. The larger the share of the fixed costs that must be paid out of each patient's bill, the more expensive the care.

Hospitals that function at low occupancy are very inefficient. Hospitals that function at high occupancy are very efficient. Having large numbers of hospitals that function at low occupancy makes for an inefficient health care system, and adds substantially to the overall cost of care.

Many cities have several hospitals, each with 50% occupancy or less, when one medium-sized hospital functioning at near capacity could provide all the hospital care for the entire city. One of the biggest problems facing the hospital industry is what to do about the oversupply of hospital beds. Few people are willing to close local hospitals. Dealing with the problem of an oversupply of hospital beds and resultant inefficiency in hospital care is a major policy challenge.

As we shall see when we discuss managed care, the effects of declining hospital occupancy are being felt throughout the country. Many hospitals have incurred large financial losses, and face the very real possibility of closing down. Hospitals began to merge to operate more efficiently. Many smaller hospitals, especially hospitals in rural areas, have had to close down completely.

Concept 3.7

The prospective payment system coupled with the movement to outpatient surgery led to a substantial decline in hospital occupancy rates. Lower occupancy rates mean less hospital income *and* a less efficient hospital. As a result many hospitals face serious financial problems.

Over the next several years there will continue to be many changes in the ownership, structure, and operation of hospitals in this country. Hardest hit by these changes will be the 1000 or so small rural hospitals that are the only health care facility available in a number of areas throughout the country, and many of the inner-city hospitals that take care of the poorest patients, most of whom rely on public support for their medical care.

Tertiary Care, Quaternary Care, and the Academic Medical Center

If primary care is provided in the physician's office and secondary care is provided either in the specialist's office or the hospital, tertiary care—the third level of care—is provided in specialized regional facilities that serve the needs of many hospitals and communities. Examples of tertiary care centers are neonatal intensive care units, burn centers, and transplant surgery centers. In many cities, each hospital has facilities for taking care of newborn babies. But when a baby is born prematurely, weighing just a fraction of what a normal baby weighs, that baby is often transferred to a hospital in the region that has developed the hugely expensive facilities and personnel necessary to provide intensive care for these neonates. Similarly, patients suffering severe burns will typically be transferred to a facility specializing in the treatment of burns.

Numerous studies have shown that when highly technical care is provided in tertiary referral centers, with a staff that frequently treats patients with those specialized needs, the outcomes for the patient are significantly better. There appears to be a strong direct relationship between the frequency with which a physician or facility performs a specialized medical procedure and the quality of the outcome for the patient. This growing awareness of the improved quality available at many tertiary referral centers has strengthened the role of these types of facilities in the era of managed care. It is at these highly specialized, tertiary referral centers that much of the training of future physicians takes place.

Concept 3.8

There appears to be a strong direct relationship between the frequency with which a physician or facility performs a specialized medical procedure and the quality of the outcome for the patient.

For some types of new, often experimental procedures, a fourth level of care has developed: quaternary care. Some facilities function as national referral centers for certain types of diseases and procedures. Examples might be combined heart and lung transplantation or experimental types of cancer treatment.

Most tertiary care centers, and nearly all quaternary care centers, are within hospitals affiliated with a university medical school. These academic medical centers fulfill a dual role. They provide most of the medical research that leads to new types of treatments, and they train the future physicians who will be applying those treatments. Academic medical centers play a crucial role in maintaining and advancing the quality of medical care in this country. Yet, in the current environment of reduced hospital occupancy and reduced payments for hospital services, even academic medical centers have been facing serious financial problems. Academic hospitals have responded to these pressures in a variety of ways, including merger, closure, and conversion to for-profit status. These changes are indicative of the magnitude of the transformation taking place in the structure of academic medical centers in the United States.

REFERENCES

Arrow K. Uncertainty and the Welfare Economics of Medical Care. *American Economic Review* 1963; 53:941–69.

Association of American Medical Colleges. U.S. Medical School Applicants Still Exceed Available Positions. www.aamc.org/newsroom/pressrel/001025.htm accessed 7/5/01.

Baker RB, Caplan AL, Emanuel LL, Latham SR. (eds.) *The American Medical Ethics Revolution—How the AMA's Code of Ethics Has Transformed Physicians' Relationships to Patients, Professionals, and Society.* Baltimore: Johns Hopkins University Press, 1999.

Flexner A. *Medical Education in the United States and Canada.* New York: Carnegie Foundation for the Advancement of Teaching, 1910.

Garfield S, Cutting C, Feldman R, et al. *Total Health Care Project Final Report.* Oakland, CA: Permanente Medical Group, 1987.

Iglehart JK. The American Health Care System—Community Hospitals. *New England Journal of Medicine* 1993; 329:372–376.

Maule WF. Screening for Colorectal Cancer by Nurse Endoscopists. *New England Journal of Medicine* 1994; 330:183–87.

Miller RS, Dunn MR, Richter TH. Graduate Medical Education, 1998–1999. *JAMA* 1999; 282:855–60.

Miller RS, Dunn MR, Richter TH, Whitcomb ME. Employment-Seeking Experiences of Resident Physicians Completing Training During 1996. *JAMA* 1998; 280:777–83.

Pasko T, Seidman B. (eds.) *Physician Characteristics and Distribution in the US.* Chicago: American Medical Association, 1999.

Salkever DS, Skinner EA, Steinwachs DM, Katz H. Episode-Based Efficiency Comparisons for Physicians and Nurse Practitioners. *Medical Care* 1982; 20(2):143–53.

Schemo DJ. Medical School Applications Dip Sharply; Minorities Rise Slightly. *New York Times,* October 27, 2000. National edition Section A, p. 18, col. 1.

Smith DB. *Health Care Divided—Race and Healing a Nation.* Ann Arbor: University of Michigan Press, 1999.

Starr P. *The Social Transformation of American Medicine.* New York: Basic Books, 1982.

United States Office of Technology Assessment. *Nurse Practitioners, Physician Assistants, and Certified Nurse-Midwives: A Policy Analysis.* Washington D.C.: United States Office of Technology Assessment, 1986.

Wennberg JE. Future Directions for Small Area Variations. *Medical Care* 1993; 31:YS75–80.

Wennberg JE, Barnes BA, Zubkoff M. Professional Uncertainty and the Problem of Supplier-Induced Demand. *Social Science and Medicine* 1982; 16:811–24.

Wennberg JE, Gittelsohn A. Small Area Variations in Health Care Delivery. *Science* 1973; 182:1102–08.

Wright RA. Community Oriented Primary Care—The Cornerstone of Health Care Reform. *JAMA* 1993; 269:2544–2547.

Zhang P, Tran SL. (eds.) *Physician Socioeconomic Statistics.* Chicago: American Medical Association, 1999.

CHAPTER 4

Paying for Health Care: Health Insurance and the Birth of the HMO

Key Concepts

- Largely as a result of two decisions by the federal government in the 1940s and 1950s, neither of which dealt specifically with health care, our country has adopted an employment-based system of financing health care. Most employees now obtain their health insurance as a nontaxable fringe benefit from work.

- The tax exclusion of health insurance obtained as a fringe benefit from work encourages employees to obtain more insurance than they would if they were paying for it themselves, often involving more comprehensive benefits and lower out-of-pocket expenditures.

- Under an *indemnity insurance plan* patients arrange care on their own and are reimbursed for the cost of the care. Reimbursement for care is financed by insurance premiums. Under a *service plan* patients come to an identified source of care and receive whatever service they need.

The cost of providing these services comes from the pooling of monthly contributions.

- *Capitation* is a method of paying for health care, under which a provider of service receives a fixed amount of money per person (the capitation rate) and in return agrees to provide all necessary care to enrolled members. Capitation rates are usually per month or per year.

- Certain types of prepaid group practice service plans are able to provide care that is substantially less expensive than traditional fee-for-service care. Health outcomes under the two systems are approximately the same. The experience of obtaining care from a prepaid group practice, however, is often less satisfactory from the patient's perspective.

- A traditional, fee-for-service insurance system has few incentives to constrain the cost of care. An HMO system has powerful incentives to constrain the cost of care.

I n looking at alternative ways to pay for health care it is important to appreciate that health care does not fit well into the traditional insurance model. Insurance is based on the concept of the random hazard: houses will burn down somewhat at random, people will get into car accidents somewhat at random. It is possible to separate people into risk categories, but within a risk category, hazards are assumed to occur somewhat randomly. One can predict the average rate at which hazards will occur within a certain risk group, estimate the aggregate cost of these hazards, add on a certain percentage for profit and administrative costs, and divide the total by the total number of people to be insured. This gives you the insurance premium to be charged.

Two aspects of health care make it particularly inappropriate for this insurance model.

1. Rather than being a truly random occurrence, the need for health care is to a large extent defined by doctors. The pattern of treatment and the associated costs of an illness or injury can vary substantially from doctor to doctor.

2. Health insurance is particularly subject to the problem of "moral hazard:" once a person is insured, that person is more likely to define a problem as an illness and is more likely to seek care.

These factors make it very difficult to predict health care expenditures for a population group. As a result, many traditional insurance companies shied away from insuring for health care. Prior to the 1930s few options were available for purchasing insurance to cover the cost of medical care. Those plans that did exist usually provided services directly to members of certain employee or other work-based groups, and were not available to the general public.

This all changed during the Great Depression of the 1930s. As discussed in Chapter 3, the inability of many individuals and families to pay the cost of medical care led to the creation of the Blue Cross and Blue Shield programs. Both the American Medical Association and the American Hospital Association supported these new plans, as long as doctors maintained control over medical decisions. By 1939, a majority of states had developed insurance programs of this type.

Federal Policies That Boosted Employee Health Insurance

Health insurance plans covered a relatively small number of people prior to World War II. However, an important decision was made in the 1940s that was to have far-reaching effects on health insurance and health care. During World War II, in order to prevent inflation, the federal government placed price controls on most consumer goods. This included a freeze on all wages. The government ruled, however, that any fringe benefits from work were exempt from price controls. Thus employees and their labor unions could not bargain for increased wages, but they could bargain for better health insurance as a fringe benefit. These policies carried over into the period after World War II, leading to greater and greater emphasis on increasing fringe benefits from work as well as wages. The main fringe benefit workers sought was health insurance.

A second government decision was to have equally powerful effects. In 1954 the government ruled that fringe benefits did not count as taxable income, and thus were not subject to income tax. The combination of these two policies has had profound effects on the way we pay for health care as a society and what we have come to expect from health care as individuals. Consider the following example, as illustrated in Figure 4.1.

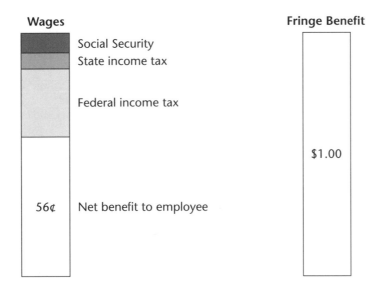

Figure 4.1 Net Benefit to Employee of $1.00 Taken Either as Added Wages or Added Fringe Benefits

If an employer wanted to raise an employee's pay by $1, the employer would have two choices: give the $1 as additional cash wages, or use the $1 to purchase additional fringe benefits. To the employer the two options are roughly equivalent, as either can be considered as a tax-deductible business expense. (The employer would have to pay certain payroll taxes on the cash contribution that would not be required for the added fringe benefits.) However, from the perspective of the worker, the two options look very different. Under tax law, the added $1 of wages would be subject to a combination of federal, state, and Social Security taxes that would, for a typical middle-income worker, eat up as much as 44¢, leaving the worker with a net gain of 56¢. On the other hand, if the worker took the added $1 as fringe benefits such as health insurance, he would get a full $1 worth of benefit, since no taxes would apply. To the worker, it is often preferable to take a wage increase as an added fringe benefit rather than as cash wages. To the employer, it makes less difference. Workers have thus come to expect to receive their health insurance as a fringe benefit of their employment.

In essence, this policy provides a federal tax subsidy for the purchase of health insurance as a fringe benefit. It is not a direct subsidy, but rather an indirect subsidy, in that less money comes into the federal treasury. This federal subsidy costs the treasury tens of billions of dollars in lost tax revenues every year and constitutes the third largest federal health care program after Medicare and Medicaid. The laws that created this subsidy were passed to address problems very different from health insurance, yet their cumulative effect over time has been to create a de facto national policy of employment-based health insurance. As is often the case, policy decisions at the federal level have long-range effects that were never envisioned at the time of their original passage.

Concept 4.1

Largely as a result of two decisions by the federal government in the 1940s and 1950s, neither of which dealt specifically with health care, our country has adopted an employment-based system of financing health care. Most employees now obtain their health insurance as a nontaxable fringe benefit from work.

A consequence of these tax policies is that people who receive health insurance as a fringe benefit tend to want more health insurance than they would if they were paying for it themselves. Consider the following example.

Assume for the moment that you are a patient with a health insurance policy with a $500 yearly deductible. (That is, you pay the first $500 for medical care each year, and the insurance policy pays 100% of everything over $500.) Assume also that you have a medical condition such as asthma, and you expect to incur at least $500 in yearly medical expenses. Finally, assume that you have $1000 in a savings account.

A friendly insurance agent offers you the following option.

- *Option 1:* The agent offers to sell you an additional health insurance policy to cover the first $500 of medical expenses each year. The cost of this policy is $600 ($500 to cover your expected medical costs, $50 to cover the administrative costs of the policy, and $50 to cover profit for the agent and the insurance company).

Do you want to buy the policy? Would any reasonable person in your situation choose to buy this policy?

It does not make much sense to purchase a policy to cover $500 in medical expenses when that policy costs $600. It makes more sense to politely refuse the insurance agent's offer and to pay the expenses directly, thus saving the $100 you would otherwise have to pay to cover overhead and profit for the insurance company. For people without a known medical condition, it makes even less sense to buy the second policy.

Your employer, it turns out, has had a very good year, and decides to give you a raise in salary of $600 per year. Now consider option 2.

- *Option 2:* The agent has heard of your good fortune, and again offers to sell you the additional health insurance policy to cover the first $500 of medical expenses each year. The cost of this policy is again $600, but the agent reasons that since you have received a raise of $600, you will now be more interested in the policy.

However, as previously illustrated in Figure 4.1, you pay 44% of any additional salary in taxes. Thus, despite your employer's generosity you only get $336 per year more in take-home pay after the raise ($600 X 56%). For the same reasons cited in option 1, it still makes no sense to buy the second policy.

- *Option 3:* Your employer, instead of giving you a raise in salary, offers to buy you the same supplemental health insurance policy to cover the first $500 in medical expenses each year. The cost of the policy to the employer is still $600.

Now do you want to buy the policy? What is the cost of the policy to you, in terms of income you have to forgo?

If you take the raise in pay as wages, you will get $336 in net benefit per year. If you take the raise as added health insurance, you will receive $500 in benefit (the $500 you would otherwise have paid out of pocket to pay for the care for your asthma). In this case, it makes sense to ask your employer to give you your raise in the form of added health insurance, even though you would never buy the same level of insurance if you were paying with your own money.

> ## Concept 4.2
>
> The tax exclusion of health insurance obtained as a fringe benefit from work encourages employees to obtain more insurance than they would if they were paying for it themselves, often involving more comprehensive benefits and lower out-of-pocket expenditures.

If you went out to purchase a car, and you were guaranteed a government subsidy for 44% of the price of a car, you would buy a very different car than you would if you had to pay the full price yourself. The same is true of health insurance. This federal policy has led to people choosing, wanting, and expecting health insurance policies that are more comprehensive than people would select for themselves if they were paying with their own money.

Based on these federal policies, employer–provided, government–subsidized private health insurance came to be the predominant model of health insurance in this country. Until the 1980s this employer-based health insurance provided in nearly all cases what has been referred to as indemnity insurance. The company indemnifies the patient for the cost of health care. The patient seeks out medical care, pays the provider directly, and in turn is reimbursed by the insurance company.

Most of these employer-provided health plans used what is called "experience rating" in determining how much to charge the employer for the cost of care. Premiums were set according to a combination of factors: the projected cost of providing care for employees, administrative costs and profit for the insurance company, and the carryover of any losses from the previous year. So long as insurance companies were able to predict accurately how much it would cost to provide medical care for all the employees each year, premiums paid by employers would rise at a gradual, predictable rate. However, if medical care costs were to rise rapidly and unpredictably, yearly increases in indemnity insurance premiums could be quite large, as illustrated in Figure 4.2.

For a period in the 1980s, this was precisely the situation confronting both employers and insurers. Due largely to the explosion in medical technology, health care costs began to rise more rapidly than anyone expected. The result was that many indemnity insurance carriers found that the actual health care costs for which they were responsible were considerably more than they had predicted, resulting in a loss for the year. This "underwriting loss" would then be added to the premiums charged to an employer for the coming year. The employer was hit with a double increase, paying

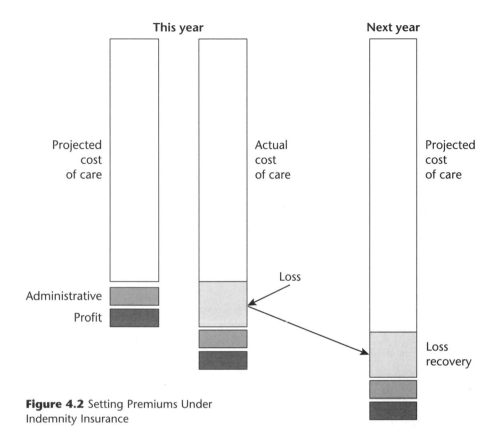

Figure 4.2 Setting Premiums Under Indemnity Insurance

for both the increase in the cost of care predicted for this year and for the underwriting loss for the previous year. Employers faced increasing costs for their employees' health insurance based on the experience of their employees during the previous year (thus the name "experience rating"). In essence the insurance company passed on to the employer the risk involved in insuring their employees for the cost of health care.

Many of the indemnity insurance companies acted mainly as pass-through agents, taking a share of all premiums to pay overhead and profit while assuming relatively little risk. A number of large companies concluded that it would be cheaper to pay for their own employees' health care directly, rather than paying an insurance company to do it for them. They established self-insurance plans that lowered administrative costs and kept the part of the premium paid to cover insurance company profit. The money that they would have paid for health insurance premiums was put aside in a special health care fund. When employees got sick, they simply gave the bill to their employer, with no insurance middleman. Many companies hired consulting firms to handle only the administration of the plan. At one point in the early 1990s, just prior to the explosion in managed care, nearly half of all employers and more than 80% of companies larger than 5000 employees provided health insurance through these self-insured plans.

However, as discussed in Chapter 1, the cost of medical care continued to rise sharply. Paying for the cost of health insurance was an increasingly large part of the cost of doing business. Insuring employees based on the indemnity model, in which most physicians and hospitals could still count on a fee for every service they performed with little oversight or constraint on the use of services, was proving to be unworkable. Thus in 1993 when President Clinton proposed a national system of care based on managed care and managed competition, many employers were initially supportive. They saw the health maintenance organizations and other managed care plans that had developed in the previous 20 years as attractive options to traditional fee-for-service, indemnity insurance.

Insurance Plans, Service Plans, and Capitation

Before discussing the origins of health maintenance organizations (HMOs) it is important first to distinguish two alternative means of providing payment for health care services and to define capitation as a method payment for health care. The traditional means of paying for health care were indemnity insurance plans, under which patients seek out their own source of care and are reimbursed for the cost of that care. Under these insurance plans, doctors were typically paid on a "fee-for-service" basis, with each separate service generating a professional fee.

As an alternative to fee-for-service medicine, a number of organizations in the early part of this century wanted to provide health care directly to a defined population of patients rather than reimbursing patients for the cost of care. These included organizations such as farm cooperatives, factories, and mining towns. Under these arrangements, a certain amount of money would be contributed each month, either by the workers or by their employer. This money would be pooled, and would be used to hire doctors to take care of the people and to pay for hospital care for the people. Each patient covered under this type of service plan was assured of the opportunity to receive all necessary medical care with no fees other than the previously established monthly contribution. Physicians working under service plans were typically paid a salary rather than on a fee-for-service basis.

Both insurance plans and service plans work on a prepaid basis. The insurance plan depends on insurance premiums, paid either by the employer or the individual employee. The service plan depends on a fixed amount of money contributed (again paid either by the employer or the

---

Concept 4.3

Under an *indemnity insurance plan* patients arrange care on their own and are reimbursed for the cost of the care. Reimbursement for care is financed by insurance premiums.

Under a *service plan* patients come to an identified source of care and receive whatever service they need. The cost of providing these services comes from pooling monthly contributions.

Concept 4.4

Capitation is a method of paying for health care, under which a provider of service receives a fixed amount of money per person (the capitation rate) and in return agrees to provide all necessary care to enrolled members. Capitation rates are usually per month or per year.

---

individual employee) to a central pool of funds. From this pool of funds, the costs of providing service to patients enrolled in the plan must be drawn. Thus for the service plan, a fixed amount of money is available for care each year. Any losses incurred cannot simply be added to the costs of next year's care. Service plans use what has come to be called the "capitation" method of paying for health care.

Throughout the early part of the twentieth century, as it was gaining increasing power over the practice of medicine, the American Medical Association (AMA) opposed the creation of service plans. The AMA objected to two aspects of service plans: doctors being paid a salary instead of fees for services, and doctors being employed by an organization rather than being independent practitioners. Even though many patients and doctors liked these arrangements, the AMA declared both of these practices to be unethical. Any doctor who violated the ethical rules established by the AMA was barred from using local community hospitals. Since these doctors couldn't use a hospital, they couldn't take care of their patients. In the face of this opposition from the AMA, by the 1930s most of these service plans had gone out of business.

There were, however, a few service plans that were able not only to survive but to prosper as an alternative to the traditional fee-for-service, insurance model. These included the Group Health Cooperative of Puget Sound in Seattle, the Health Insurance Plan of New York, and the Kaiser-Permanente Health Care System on the West Coast. We examine the origins of Kaiser-Permanente, the most successful of these service plans, to understand more about why these plans not only survived but eventually provided the model around which the entire movement to managed care was centered.

Kaiser-Permanente and the Development of Health Maintenance Organizations

In 1932 the City of Los Angeles began work on what was then a mammoth construction project: a 242-mile-long aqueduct across the southern California desert to bring water from the Colorado River to the growing metropolis of Los Angeles. A number of industrialists collaborated on the project, among them Henry J. Kaiser. With more than 5000 workers in the field, and with on-the-job injuries all too frequent, there was a pressing need to provide medical care for workers close to the construction site.

Sydney Garfield was a young physician who had just completed training as a surgeon at Los Angeles County Hospital. With meager prospects for employment during the depth of the Great Depression, he saw an opportunity for an independent medical practice in the desert, close to the construction sites. Borrowing $50,000, he built a small hospital and set up a traditional fee-for-service practice in the desert. Unfortunately, he soon found the income from such a practice to be much less than he expected, and his hospital was near bankruptcy (Smillie 1991).

Garfield met with a representative of Kaiser's construction company. The construction company did not want the hospital to close, as it was the only source of care close to the construction site. The two of them worked out a plan under which the company would pay Garfield $1.50 per worker per month, and in return Garfield would provide all necessary medical care for on-the-job injuries. In addition, workers were offered the opportunity of having an additional $1.50 taken out of their paychecks each month, in return for which they could go to Garfield for treatment of medical problems not related to their work. Henry Kaiser enthusiastically approved, and the plan was put in place.

This capitation arrangement offered workers a service plan rather than a traditional insurance plan and turned out to be very successful. In a short period of time the hospital was on firm financial ground and Garfield was receiving a good income.

In 1938 Henry Kaiser received the contract to build the Grand Coulee Dam on the Columbia River in eastern Washington. This construction project was far enough away from cities that many workers brought their families with them. Garfield and Kaiser agreed to establish a service plan for medical care for the workers as well as their families, based on the success-ful model in the California desert. For a fixed fee per person per month, paid partially by Kaiser and partially by the workers, employees and their fami-lies could receive all necessary care at the hospital and medical offices organ-ized by Garfield. Again the plan was successful, with Garfield hiring a num-ber of young physicians to work for his new medical plan. The labor unions representing the construction workers were especially pleased, as previous attempts at providing medical care had been of questionable quality.

Recall, however, that the American Medical Association had declared prepaid service plans based on capitation for workers and salaries for doc-tors to be unethical. An editorial published in the *Journal of the American Medical Association* in 1932 labeled these prepaid group practice plans "med-ical soviets" and went on to say that, "such plans will mean the destruction of private practice . . . they are, in a word, 'unethical'" (American Medical Association 1932). However, since both the Los Angeles aqueduct project and the Grand Coulee project were in rural areas, the AMA and their local affiliates paid little attention to them. Also, since Garfield operated his own hospital close to the work sites, he didn't need to have medical society approval to use a hospital. World War II, however, was to change all of this.

When World War II came, Kaiser quickly began producing liberty ships at shipyards in Portland, Oregon, and in Richmond, California. Much of the steel for these ships came from the Kaiser steel mill in southern California. Again Henry Kaiser turned to Garfield to organize the medical care for ship-yard workers and their families. This time the AMA and its state affiliates opposed the plan and would not permit Dr. Garfield or the more than 90 doctors he had hired to use local hospitals. Despite a personal visit by Henry Kaiser to its Chicago headquarters, the AMA would not relent. Faced with no alternative, Kaiser either built or bought a hospital in each of the three locales where the new Kaiser health plan was in operation.

After World War II, many employee groups beyond the shipyard work-ers wanted to join Kaiser's health plan. It provided a guarantee of all nec-essary care for a fixed fee per month. People liked both the price and the guaranteed availability of care. The AMA, however, continued to oppose Kaiser and other prepaid group practices. Through a series of legal actions in the 1940s and 1950s, the organized medical profession aggressively tried to put these plans out of business. Based largely on antitrust laws, the health plans were able to gain court protections, and in the late 1950s a truce of sorts was achieved. The AMA ended its efforts to close the Kaiser Health Plan.

The Kaiser plan grew and became very successful due largely to its suc-cess with labor unions and other large employee groups. Unfortunately, this growth and success contributed to tension between Henry Kaiser and

Garfield. Each wanted to control the growing organization. After lengthy negotiations they agreed to maintain three separate organizations: a health plan, a hospitals corporation, and a doctors' group. Kaiser would be in charge of the hospital and health plan organizations. Garfield would be in charge of the doctors' organization. Kaiser agreed that he would use only Garfield's doctor organization for the patients covered by his health plan. Garfield agreed that his doctors would treat only patients in Kaiser's health plan. Thus, they were each dependent on the other.

The resulting Kaiser-Permanente Health Plan grew and prospered throughout the 1950s and '60s. It consistently cost less than comparable care under fee-for-service insurance. From its original three hospitals, it grew to become the largest HMO in the United States, providing care in several regions of the country. It depended on the continued cooperation and interdependence of the physicians, the hospitals, and the health plan. The health plan was set up as a nonprofit foundation plan, allowing it to remain tax-exempt. Likewise the hospitals were owned and operated by a nonprofit corporation. Only the doctors operated on a for-profit basis. The structure of the Kaiser-Permanente Health Plan is illustrated in Figure 4.3.

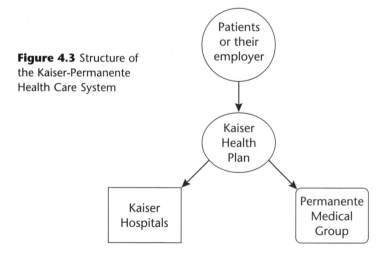

Figure 4.3 Structure of the Kaiser-Permanente Health Care System

As discussed above, the model represented by Kaiser-Permanente and other similar plans was called "prepaid group practice." For a fixed monthly fee (the capitation rate) paid to the Kaiser Foundation Health Plan either by patients or their employer, the Health Plan would provide its members with all necessary health care. They would do this by contracting with the Kaiser hospital corporation for hospital care and with the Permanente Medical Group for physician care and other outpatient services.

The service plans represented by prepaid group practices such as Kaiser-Permanente were consistently able to provide comprehensive care at a substantially lower cost than the insurance plans using the traditional fee-for-service method of paying for care. Repeated research studies documented this fact. However, critics of these plans suggested that their lower cost of care was because they tended to attract younger, healthier patients who needed less care. If they took care of comparable patient populations, it was suggested, their cost advantage would disappear.

This issue was settled convincingly by a study done by the Rand Corporation in the 1980s (Manning et al. 1984). The Rand Health Insurance Experiment enrolled a group of 1580 patients in Seattle and paid for their health insurance for a period of between three and five years. In order to be sure that patients in one type of system weren't sicker on average than the other, the study randomly assigned patients either to receive all care from the Group Health Cooperative of Puget Sound (a large, prepaid group practice similar in many ways to Kaiser-Permanente) or from traditional fee-for-service physician offices. The results of this study are shown in Table 4.1.

Table 4.1   Comparison of the Annual Cost of Care Under Prepaid Group Practice and Fee-for-Service Systems

System	Total Cost per Patient	Hospital Admissions per 1000 Patients	Office Visits per Patient
HMO	$439	8.4	4.3
Fee-for-service	$609	13.8	4.2

Source: Manning et al. 1984

This study demonstrated that, given comparable patient populations, prepaid group practice service plans could be as much as one-third less expensive than fee-for-service insurance plans for comparable care.

The researchers also studied whether patients' health was any better in one type of plan or the other. Poor people in the prepaid group practice tended to have problems in two areas—blood pressure control and control of glaucoma. Otherwise the health of the two groups of patients was substantially the same (Sloss et al 1987).

It is important to point out that the difference between prepaid group practice and fee-for-service systems in this study was in the use of hospitals, and not in the use of outpatient physician services. There was no evidence that the use of primary care services and other outpatient services was different in prepaid group practices compared to fee-for-service.

However, patients found the experience of obtaining care from the pre-paid group practices to be significantly less satisfactory than from the fee-for-service system (Davies et al. 1986). As shown in Table 4.2, patient satisfaction was lower for a number of aspects of the primary care process.

Table 4.2   Comparison of Patient Satisfaction with Prepaid Group Practice (PPGP) and Fee-for-Service (FFS) Systems

Differences in Mean Satisfaction ($p < .05$)

Satisfaction With:	PPGP	FFS
Access to care	–	+
Waiting time in the office	+	–
Technical quality of care	NS	NS
Interpersonal nature of care	–	+
Overall satisfaction with care	–	+

Source: Davies et al. 1986
Note: Lower satisfaction indicated by –, higher satisfaction by +, no significant difference by NS. $p < .05$

Concept 4.5

Certain types of prepaid group practice service plans are able to provide care that is substantially less expensive than traditional fee-for-service care. Health outcomes under the two systems are approximately the same. The experience of obtaining care from a prepaid group practice, however, is often less satisfactory from the patient's perspective.

The HMO Act of 1973 and the Expansion of HMOs

Even prior to the Rand Health Insurance Experiment, a number of individuals and groups, both within government and in the private sector, had taken note of the cost savings available through prepaid group practice service plans. Several leaders of organized labor, led by Walter Reuther of the United Auto Workers Union, called for national health care reform based on expansion of the prepaid group practice model. In 1970 Senator Edward Kennedy introduced legislation to this end, setting off a national debate about health care reform.

Even at that time many states still had laws making prepaid group practice illegal. These laws were left over from the period when the AMA was fighting against the growth of prepaid group practice.

A number of groups introduced proposals for reform. Although Congress was not able to agree on comprehensive reform, it did pass the Health Maintenance Organizations Act of 1973 (P.L.93-222). Following the enactment of this law, prepaid group practices came to be known instead as health maintenance organizations, or simply HMOs. The HMO Act did five main things.

1. It removed preexisting state laws inhibiting HMOs.

2. It offered federal subsidies for the establishment of new, nonprofit HMOs.

3. It defined minimum standards to be certified as a "federally qualified HMO." A key element of these standards was the requirement that the HMO be organized on a nonprofit basis.

4. Where HMOs were available, it required all employers who offered health insurance to their employees to also offer an HMO as an option.

5. In a compromise with the American Medical Association, it broadened the definition of an HMO to include a fee-for-service option, referred to as an independent practice association or IPA.

Thus there were three basic models on which HMOs could function. Each is a service plan in that patients receive service from an established list of physicians without receiving a bill. Each functions under the capitation method of payment, meaning that there is a fixed budget each year from which all necessary services must be paid for. The three basic options for early HMO development are described below.

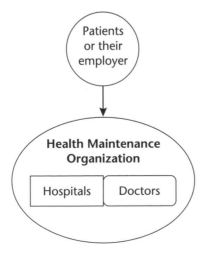

Figure 4.4 Staff Model HMO

In a staff model HMO, illustrated in Figure 4.4, the HMO owns the hospital and employs the doctors. The doctors are paid a fixed salary, with no financial incentive to provide more care. The hospital operates under a fixed annual budget, needing to manage the use of resources so as to have adequate funds remaining at the end of the yearly budget cycle. Patients or their employers make the capitation payment directly to the HMO, and receive care only from the physicians and hospitals of the HMO. The Group Health Cooperative of Puget Sound is an example of a staff model HMO.

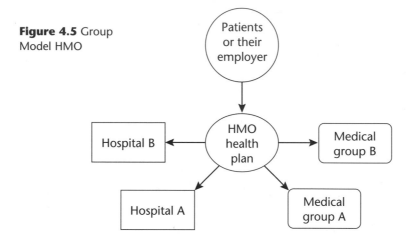

Figure 4.5 Group Model HMO

In a group model HMO, illustrated in Figure 4.5, the HMO operates a health plan that does not provide care directly. It owns no hospitals and hires no doctors. Instead it contracts with groups of doctors to provide care to its members and with either a chain of hospitals or a series of individual hospitals to provide hospital care for its members. The physician groups in turn are paid a subcapitation rate from the HMO. Through a contract with the HMO the medical group is paid a share of the capitation rate received by the HMO and agrees in return to provide all necessary physician services for the members of the HMO who select that medical group for their care. Within each medical group, doctors can be paid either by salary, a fixed annual fee for each patient cared for, or fee-for-service, depending on how the group is organized internally. Hospitals can be paid either a fixed amount per year or separately for each hospital admission.

An independent practice association HMO is a corporation usually formed and managed by physicians locally. The HMO accepts capitation payments for enrolled members and in turn contracts with individual doctors who have signed a contract with the IPA, illustrated in Figure 4.6. Under the contract the doctor agrees to treat HMO patients either on a dis-

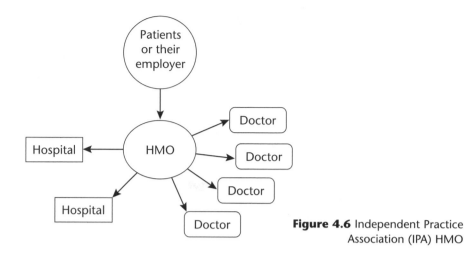

Figure 4.6 Independent Practice Association (IPA) HMO

counted fee-for-service basis or in return for a fixed amount per patient per year. Hospitals that contract with the HMO are paid per admission, usually on a discounted basis.

The IPA model HMO looks a lot like the traditional fee-for-service system. Allowing the IPA model was the concession that Congress made to the AMA in 1973 in order to get the HMO Act passed. There is, however, a key difference between fee-for-service insurance plans and all types of HMOs, including the IPA. Under traditional fee-for-service plans there is no limit on how much can be spent on care each year. For all types of HMOs, a fixed amount of money is available each year based on the capitation rate and the number of members enrolled. An HMO is obligated to provide all necessary care to all enrolled members for that amount of money.

In a fee-for-service indemnity insurance system, there is no incentive to hold down costs:

- Not for the patient, who only pays a small amount of the actual bill

- Not for the hospitals, which get paid for each patient regardless of how necessary the care is

- Not for doctors, whose incentive is to provide more care, since the more care they provide the more money they get

- Not for the insurance company, because if it loses money in a given year it simply adds that loss onto the insurance rates for the next year

In an HMO, on the other hand, there is a strong incentive to hold down costs. An excessive use of services early in the year can lead to a budget shortfall later in the year, leaving inadequate funds to cover salaries and other costs. Physicians in an HMO must be careful to provide only that care that is absolutely necessary. As we saw from the Rand Health Insurance

Experiment, the incentives in an HMO to hold down costs have been associated with cost savings of more than 30% relative to the fee-for-service alternative. These savings were mainly in the use of the hospital and other expensive, high-tech treatments and not in the use of primary care and other outpatient services.

> ## Concept 4.6
>
> A traditional, fee-for-service insurance system has few incentives to constrain the cost of care. An HMO system has powerful incentives to constrain the cost of care.

Other Types of Managed Care Plans

Since the enactment of the HMO Act of 1973 a variety of new managed care plans have been developed to compete both with HMOs and with traditional fee-for-service systems. These new plans use many of the same mechanisms to reduce utilization and costs, but they are more loosely structured than HMOs and they don't technically qualify as HMOs. Several of these plans are described below.

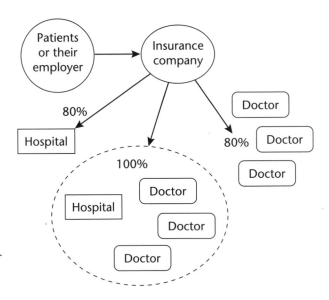

Figure 4.7 Preferred Provider Organization (PPO)

A preferred provider organization (PPO) is usually organized by an insurance company as an alternative to traditional indemnity insurance.

The insurance company contracts with a group of doctors and hospitals that agree to give a discount to patients with this insurance. These providers are called preferred providers. A patient with this type of insurance can go anywhere for care, but if the patient chooses a doctor or a hospital not on the list of preferred providers, the patient has to pay substantially more for care. For example, the PPO might pay 100% of the cost of care from preferred providers and only 80% of the cost of care from other providers (see Figure 4.7). There is usually some form of control over the use of hospital treatment in PPOs, but it is not as stringent as in an HMO. The doctors in a PPO have no financial stake in the success of the company.

A point of service plan (POS) is a hybrid plan that includes elements of both an HMO and a PPO. Patients in a POS plan have three choices for receiving care, each with a different level of coverage.

1. If the patient receives care from doctors in the HMO, the patient pays very little for care (usually on the level of $5–10 per visit).
2. If the patient receives care from doctors on the list of preferred providers associated with the POS, the patient pays a larger portion of the cost of care (typically 20% of the cost of care).
3. If the patient receives care from a doctor or hospital not associated with the POS, the patient pays a substantial portion of the cost of care (typically 40–50%).

Thus in a POS the member has three options for obtaining care (see Figure 4.8). The more the member is willing to limit his choice of physicians to those in the HMO or contracting with the POS, the less the member has

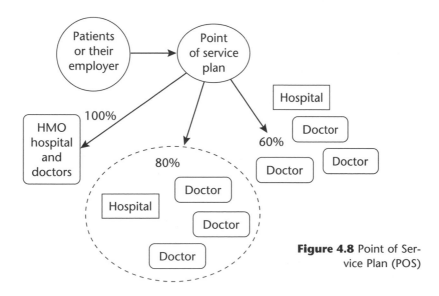

Figure 4.8 Point of Service Plan (POS)

to pay. Because of this ability to choose the level of coverage, POS plans are sometimes referred to as "triple option plans."

In a number of areas of the country, groups of physicians have banded together with local hospitals to form their own local health care plans, referred to as physician-hospital organizations (PHOs). They usually work with large employers to offer this plan to employees as an alternative to HMOs. As discussed in Chapter 7, a number of the larger HMOs have evolved into essentially middlemen, accepting capitation payments from employers and passing the capitation payments along to physicians and hospitals (after keeping a portion of the payment for profit and administrative overhead). A PHO is intended to cut out the middleman, and to have capitation payments made directly to physicians and hospitals working together.

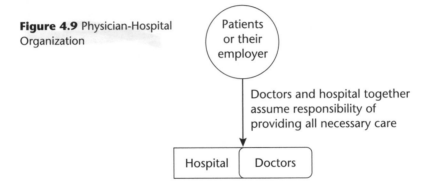

Figure 4.9 Physician-Hospital Organization

Patients or their employer

Doctors and hospital together assume responsibility of providing all necessary care

Hospital | Doctors

A PHO does not involve an insurance company or health plan directly. The doctors agree to provide all necessary physician care and the hospital agrees to provide all necessary hospital care to all patients enrolled in the plan (see Figure 4.9). If a type of sub-specialist physician is not available in the doctors' group, or if a type of hospital service is not available at the hospital, then the PHO must arrange to pay for this care at another institution, without charging the member anything in addition to the usual premium.

The advantage of the PHO is that it maintains local control over medical decisions, with no insurance company setting arbitrary treatment policies that the doctors must follow. The potential disadvantage of this type of plan is the difficulty of ensuring the financial security of the plan. It takes a large plan with several hundred physicians and more than one hospital to have sufficient financial resources to absorb the extraordinary costs that come from taking care of critically ill patients, such as those requiring organ transplantation. If the plan is not sufficiently large, and if it then faces these extraordinary expenses, it risks running out of money and being unable to fulfill its obligation to provide all necessary care for its members.

It is interesting to note that PHOs that are being developed as alternatives to HMOs are very similar in structure to the original structure of the Kaiser-Permanente system. The very model that for years was anathema to most physicians is becoming, for many of them, a principal alternative to HMOs and other types of newer health plans owned and operated by large, for-profit corporations.

The cost savings of HMOs documented by the Rand Health Insurance Experiment pertain to large, centralized HMOs such as Kaiser-Permanente and Group Health Cooperative of Puget Sound. The structure of many of the newer HMOs, especially IPAs, is quite different from the traditional model with salaried doctors and centralized facilities. It was not known if many of the newer types of HMOs are able to achieve the same cost savings compared to fee-for-service systems. To answer this question another large study was undertaken: the Medical Outcomes Study (Safran et al. 1994). This study involved 1208 patients with chronic disease, followed for four years. The patients were enrolled in one of three types of plan: a large group model HMO, an IPA HMO, and a traditional fee-for-service indemnity plan. The study followed two main outcomes: primary care quality and the change in patients' health status over the four years of the study. Results of the study for primary care quality, comparing the three alternative systems, are shown in Table 4.3.

Table 4.3   Primary Care Quality in a Group HMO, IPA HMO, and Fee-for-Service System: Medical Outcomes Study

	HMO	IPA	FFS
Cost of care	++	+	−
Coordination	+	−	−
Access to care	−	+	+
Comprehensiveness	−	+	+
Continuity	−	+	++
Doctor's interpersonal skills	NS	NS	NS
Doctor's technical skills	NS	NS	NS

Source: Safran et al. 1994.

Note: Results show comparative levels of quality, from − (low) to ++ (highest). NS = no significant difference.

$p < .05$

Compared to the IPA HMO and the fee-for-service option, the group HMO had a lower cost of care and better coordination among specialists and primary care doctors. However, it had lower ratings than either alternative for access to care, continuity of care, and comprehensiveness of care. There were no significant differences in how patients viewed either the interpersonal or the technical skills of their doctors. Overall there were no significant differences in health outcomes for the patients studied, although low-income patients did show worse health outcomes in the group HMO.

These findings are quite similar to the findings of the Rand experiment: although HMOs save money, they have problems in the quality of the primary care process. These problems frequently lead to lower overall levels of patient satisfaction in HMOs compared to a fee-for-service system. IPA HMOs, which rely on fee-for-service payment to physicians under an overall capitated framework, seem to fall somewhere between group HMOs and traditional fee-for-service. In addition, these studies consistently identify worse health outcomes for low-income patients enrolled in HMOs. The causes of these poorer health outcomes are not fully understood, although they may have to do with low-income patients having problems navigating the complex organizational systems inherent in many large HMOs.

By the early 1990s the accumulated evidence showed that HMOs and other types of managed care plans offered a way to reduce the cost of care without adverse effects on the health of most patients. The federal government, state governments, and employers began to look at them as alternatives to traditional fee-for-service care. The growing popularity of these plans set the stage for the dramatic shifts in health care delivery sparked by the national debate on health care reform that followed the election of President Clinton, as discussed in Chapter 7.

REFERENCES

American Medical Association. The Committee on the Costs of Medical Care (editorial). *JAMA* 1932; 99:1950

Davies AR, Ware JE, Brook RH, et al. Consumer Acceptance of Prepaid and Fee-for-Service Medical Care: Results from a Randomized Controlled Trial. *Health Services Research* 1986; 21:429–49.

Manning WG, Leibowitz A, Goldberg GA, et al. A Controlled Trial of the Effect of a Prepaid Group Practice on Use of Services. *New England Journal of Medicine* 1984; 310:1505–10.

Safran D, Tarlov AR, Rogers WH. Primary Care Performance in Fee-for-Service and Prepaid Health Systems. *JAMA* 1994; 271:1579–86.

Sloss EM, Keeler EB, Brook RH, et al. Effect of a Health Maintenance Organization on Physiologic Health. *Annals of Internal Medicine* 1987; 106:130–38.

Smillie JG. *Can Physicians Manage the Quality and Costs of Health Care? The Story of the Permanente Medical Group*. New York: McGraw-Hill, 1991.

CHAPTER 5

Medicare

Key Concepts

- As a result of a last-minute political compromise, the federal Medicare program was designed as a combination service plan (Part A) and insurance plan (Part B).

- The Medicare program has today's workers pay the costs of today's retirees. The number of active workers per beneficiary is projected to decline from 3.9 in 1998 to 2.3 in 2030.

- About 75 cents out of every dollar spent on Medicare Part B comes out of general tax revenues.

- Only 13% of Medicare beneficiaries have coverage limited to Medicare. The other 87% of beneficiaries obtain a supplemental "medigap" policy to cover costs not paid by Medicare.

- The resource-based relative value scale (RBRVS) established a simplified method for paying physicians treating Medicare patients. Instituting the scale improved the equity in the way primary care physicians and procedural specialists are paid, and provided a mechanism for controlling overall Part B Medicare costs.

- Medicare spends most of its money taking care of a very few people: the care of 23% of the elderly population uses 85% of Medicare funds.

- The administrative structure of Medicare, managed by the federal Health Care Financing Administration, is the most efficient medical payment system in the country.

The facsimile of a pay stub, in Figure 5.1, a typical one for students who might work part-time in a college or university dining hall, offers a statement of the extent to which workers and employers are currently paying for government programs in health care. Of the five categories of withholding taxes shown on the pay stub, three go, at least in part, to pay for such programs.

The federal Medicare program, which is our system of universal health insurance for all those 65 years old or older, is paid for out of both the Medicare withholding tax and the general federal withholding tax (shown

Figure 5.1 Sample Paycheck Stub

Statement of Earnings and Taxes University Office of Dining Services		
Employee: XXXXXX XXXXXX	**Social Security No.** 999-99-9999	

Hours:
  Overtime   10.70
  Regular   78.60
Total gross
	Amount:
	89.88
	440.16
	530.04	

Gross pay: 530.04	**Taxes** 115.19	**Net pay:** 414.85

Taxes deducted:
  FICA/OAS   32.86
  Medicare   7.69
  Fed tax   63.26
  State tax   6.61
  VDI   4.77
Total tax: 115.19		

on the check as Fed tax). The Medicaid program (discussed in the following chapter), which is a federal/state partnership to provide medical insurance to the poor and disabled, is paid for out of a combination of federal taxes and state taxes (shown as State tax).

Even though every worker contributes to paying the cost of these programs, only a minority of people in this country are covered by them. In contrast to most other countries, which have adopted universal health insurance for all their citizens, the United States has pursued a policy of incrementalism: establishing government-funded programs for specific populations felt to be most vulnerable. The two largest groups benefiting from this incremental approach to national health care are the elderly and the poor. Both programs were established in 1965 after decades of debate about the proper role of government in paying for health care.

During the administration of Franklin Roosevelt, as part of the social programs enacted under his New Deal, proposals for comprehensive medical insurance were considered but ultimately abandoned in the face of overriding opposition from the American Medical Association (AMA) and other groups within the medical profession. Following World War II President Harry Truman again proposed a program of national health insurance, but again the opposition of the medical profession blocked the proposal. It was only under the unique circumstances in the mid-1960s of a Democratic president, a strongly Democratic Congress, and a national momentum for social reform that the federal government was able finally to overcome the opposition of the medical profession and enact the Medicare and Medicaid programs. (FICA/OAS is the Social Security Program, formally the Federal Insurance Contributions Act that funds Old Age, Survivors, and Disability Insurance. VDI is Voluntary Disability Insurance.)

Medicare: Universal Health Insurance for the Elderly

Medicare is the federal program that helps to pay for health care for the elderly in this country. All people 65 years of age or older who qualify for Social Security are automatically eligible for Medicare. Rather than being a separate law, Medicare was enacted as an amendment to the existing Social Security law. It is thus often referred to as Title XVIII.

At the time of the passage of Medicare in 1965, only 56% of the elderly had hospital insurance. The costs of treating a serious illness were seen as a very real threat to the financial security of seniors. There was a strong national consensus that none of the elderly in our country should face financial ruin due to illness. Medicare was the way to ensure this outcome.

As discussed in Chapter 4, there are two general types of health plans: a service plan, in which all participants are provided with a given level of service, and an insurance plan, in which participants receive reimbursement for the cost of services. The initial proposal was to create a service plan covering hospital care. Under this type of plan, the elderly would simply go to the hospital as needed, and the hospital would get paid directly by the government.

The AMA was opposed to the service plan concept. If Medicare was to be passed at all the AMA wanted it established as an insurance plan covering both hospital care and the care provided by doctors, with patients paying for care directly and getting reimbursed by the government insurance program. The AMA also wanted to keep the government out of running the program; they preferred that it be run by private insurance companies.

A last-minute compromise was struck that incorporated both proposals. Under the compromise, Medicare became a combined service and insurance program (Ball 1995). The structure of the original Medicare program is illustrated in Figure 5.2.

Concept 5.1

As a result of a last-minute political compromise, the federal Medicare program was designed as a combination service plan (Part A) and insurance plan (Part B).

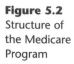

Figure 5.2
Structure of
the Medicare
Program

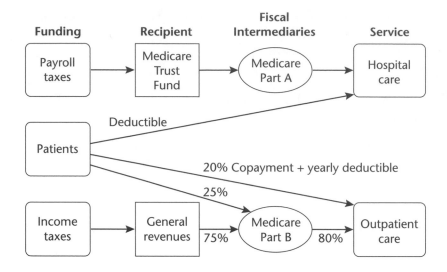

Medicare Part A

Medicare Part A is a service plan for hospital care. All eligible patients receive any necessary hospital care, paid for by the government. The patient is responsible for a deductible payment equal roughly to the cost of the first day of hospitalization. (In 1998 this amount was $764.) After this deductible amount all the costs of hospitalization are paid by Medicare for up to 60 days in the hospital per illness. If the patient needs more time in the hospital than this, the patient is responsible for $191 per day for additional days up to a maximum of 90 days' hospitalization per illness.

Medicare Part A also pays for up to 20 days in a skilled nursing facility following hospitalization, so long as the care is necessary to continue the healing or rehabilitation process. (For those patients who need to spend time in a nursing home simply because they cannot care for themselves, but are not undergoing an active treatment program, Medicare provides no payment whatsoever. These patients are referred to as receiving "custodial care" as contrasted to "skilled nursing care." The problems associated with custodial care and other types of long-term care are discussed in Chapter 9.)

Until 1997, Medicare Part A also paid for home health care. This is medically necessary care provided in the patient's home, involving such services as nursing care, physical therapy, or occupational therapy. These services are provided by Medicare-certified home health agencies on the prescription of the treating physician. Because of the rising cost of the home health care benefit and the growing realization that it was not particularly effective in its intended purpose of keeping patients out of the hospital, in 1997 the costs of home health care were transferred to the Medicare Part B budget.

Finally, Medicare Part A pays for hospice care for the terminally ill. Enacted in the 1980s as an amendment to the original Medicare legislation, the Medicare hospice program pays for extra services during the last six months of a patient's life as long as the patient is certified by a physician as terminally ill (i.e., not likely to survive more than six months) and the patient agrees to forgo aggressive treatment measures such as surgery or intensive care.

All the money to pay for Medicare Part A comes from a roughly 1.5% payroll tax levied on all workers. (On the pay stub in Figure 5.1, the tax labeled "Medicare" goes purely to finance Part A.) For every dollar in tax paid by employees, the employer is required to pay an additional dollar. The money from these taxes is deposited into the Medicare Trust Fund, essentially a savings account established by the federal government to pay hospital bills when they come in.

The government doesn't actually pay bills submitted by hospitals. Instead the government contracts with private companies to accept the bills from the hospitals and write the checks to them. The companies, referred to as "fiscal intermediaries," are then reimbursed from the Medicare Trust Fund. The creation of the fiscal intermediary was part of the compromise struck with the AMA at the time of the original passage of the Medicare legislation.

One point is important to establish at this time. The money paid in payroll taxes into the Medicare Trust Fund is not put aside to pay for the care of current workers when they retire. Instead it is used to pay for the care of people already retired. The financing of the Medicare program is based on the concept that current workers pay the medical care costs of those currently retired. When today's workers are retired, their care will be paid for by those who are working at that time. Medical care during the retirement of the baby boom generation will therefore be financed by the substantially smaller number of people born after the baby boom.

About 90% of all Medicare funds come from people currently working. In order for the system to work, there have to be enough workers paying enough taxes to pay for the care needed by the elderly. In 1998 there were 39 million beneficiaries with 153 million workers to support them, or about one beneficiary for every 3.9 workers. In 2030 as the last baby boomer turns 65, there will be an estimated 76 million beneficiaries with 177 million workers to support them. This means that for every beneficiary in 2030 there will be only about 2.3 workers. The ratio will continue to decline until there are only 2 workers per beneficiary by 2070 (data from HCFA). If the cost of care per beneficiary remains relatively constant, the tax burden on each worker will increase by nearly 70% in the next 30 years. If the cost per beneficiary goes up (as it is almost certain to do), the tax burden will increase even more. This policy dilemma inherent in the current Medicare program is one of the most pressing aspects of the forces that threaten the long-term financial viability of Medicare.

> ## Concept 5.2
>
> The Medicare program looks to today's workers to pay the costs of today's retirees. The number of active workers per beneficiary is projected to decline from 3.9 in 1998 to 2.3 in 2030.

Medicare Part B

Part B pays for doctor bills and other medical care costs that are incurred on an outpatient basis (that is, that take place outside the hospital). Under Part B, patients going to doctors, laboratories, X ray offices, and other outpatient providers of care receive a bill for each service provided. As with Part A, private companies acting as the fiscal intermediary handle all paperwork and pay out all the funds. The government acts to hold the moneys collected, and to transfer it to the fiscal intermediaries as needed.

As an insurance plan, Part B involves an insurance premium paid by the beneficiaries. This premium is withheld from the Social Security checks of all those participating in the plan, so there is no need to bill patients for the cost of the premium. In addition, Part B is voluntary; only those seniors electing to have the premium deducted from their check are covered. (This is in contrast to Part A, which is compulsory for all seniors receiving Social Security.) Nearly all seniors select Part B coverage.

The original intent for Part B was to have the premiums collected from the patients cover about half the cost of the program, with the other half of the cost coming out of general tax revenues. It rapidly became apparent that this 50/50 cost sharing was going to be too expensive for seniors to bear, so over time the premium was reduced substantially. In 1998 the Part B premium was $43.80 per month, which was sufficient to cover about 25% of the cost of the program. Thus about 75 cents out of every dollar spent on Part B comes out of general tax revenues.

> ## Concept 5.3
>
> About 75 cents out of every dollar spent on Medicare Part B comes out of general tax revenues.

Medicare Part B has two mechanisms to pay for care by physicians and other outpatient providers. They are referred to as the provider "accepting assignment" and "not accepting assignment." The choice is up to the provider (not the patient), and will affect the amount and the manner of payment for services. For both options, the patient is responsible for paying a yearly deductible of $100.

Under the first option, illustrated in Figure 5.3, the doctor (or other provider) agrees to accept an amount set by Medicare as payment in full for the service provided. (See the section below on the resource-based relative value system for an indication of how these amounts are set.) In return for the doctor setting his fee at this level, Medicare will pay the doctor directly an amount equal to 80% of that fee. The patient then is responsible for paying the doctor only the remaining 20% of the fee. Doctors and other providers who agree to accept assignment are referred to as "participating providers."

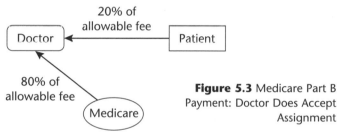

Figure 5.3 Medicare Part B Payment: Doctor Does Accept Assignment

However, the fee allowed by Medicare is usually much lower than the fee a doctor charges his other patients for the same service. Medicare fees typically are about two-thirds of the fees paid by private insurers. About half of all physicians have elected not to accept assignment, so they can charge Medicare patients a higher fee. In this case, illustrated in Figure 5.4, the patient is responsible for paying the doctor directly for the full amount billed. The patient may then send a form into Medicare and be reimbursed for 80% of Medicare's allowable fee.

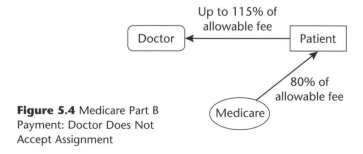

Figure 5.4 Medicare Part B Payment: Doctor Does Not Accept Assignment

In order to protect Medicare beneficiaries from having to pay extremely high doctors' fees, a law was enacted that limits the amount any physician can charge to a Medicare beneficiary to 115% of Medicare's allowable fee. Thus, if the allowable Medicare fee for a service is $100, the most a doctor may charge a Medicare patient is $115.

Even with this limitation, the fees paid by Medicare patients to doctors and other providers can be quite high. The patient is responsible for 20% of the fee to begin with; going to a doctor who does not accept assignment will add another 15%. Thus, even though they are covered by Part B insurance, patients can be required to pay 35% of all doctor bills out of pocket. (This is in addition to the $100 yearly deductible.) Consider that in 1998, two-thirds of all elderly households in the United States had total annual incomes under $21,000, and it is easy to see that out-of-pocket expenses for medical care can be a substantial burden on Medicare beneficiaries. For these families and individuals, 35% of their household income can go for health care.

A number of people in the country and in Congress want to get away from any limit on the amount that doctors can charge their Medicare patients. Legislation has been proposed that would allow "private contracting" between the doctor and the patient, whereby the doctor and patient could agree to any fee schedule they want. Such a change would essentially allow doctors to charge Medicare patients whatever they wish. (These proposals are very closely tied to the "balance billing" issue that was so hotly debated as part of the Canadian health care plan.)

Medigap Insurance

As discussed above, patients covered by Medicare are still responsible for paying a number of different costs. These include

- The Part A hospital deductible for each time they are in the hospital,
- The yearly Part B $100 deductible
- 20% of all charges covered by Part B
- The extra charges (up to 15% of allowable charges) of doctors who don't accept assignment

In addition, a number of key services are not covered at all by Medicare, including

- Prescription drugs
- Dental care
- Eyeglasses

- Hearing aids
- Foot care

In order to gain coverage for these items, 87% of Medicare beneficiaries obtain a private, supplemental insurance policy, referred to as a "medigap" policy. As the name suggests, a medigap policy is a medical insurance policy that pays for these gaps in Medicare coverage. There are three principal ways for beneficiaries to obtain medigap coverage.

1. The beneficiary can purchase the policy from a private insurance company (as 30% of Medicare beneficiaries do).
2. The beneficiary can obtain the policy from a former employer as a retirement benefit (32% of beneficiaries).
3. If the beneficiary has an income that is below the federal poverty level, the Medicaid program will provide the medigap coverage (17% of beneficiaries).

An additional 8% of beneficiaries will obtain medigap coverage in some other way, leaving only 13% of Medicare beneficiaries with coverage limited to that provided by Medicare.

Concept 5.4

Only 13% of Medicare beneficiaries have coverage limited to Medicare. The other 87% of beneficiaries obtain a supplemental "medigap" policy to cover costs not paid by Medicare.

Each medigap supplemental insurance plan will have its own set of covered benefits. Most will pay for the Part A hospital deductible, the Part B yearly deductible, and the 20% share of providers' bills not covered by Medicare. Many will also provide some coverage of prescription drugs.

The cost of these medigap policies has been increasing substantially in recent years. After several years of yearly premium increases in the range of 3–6%, in the late 1990s medigap policies began to go up by as much as 10–20% per year. In addition, the rapid escalation in the cost of prescription drugs made this coverage option unaffordable for many beneficiaries. Premium increases have placed a substantial burden on a number of Medicare beneficiaries, and have encouraged many of them to enroll in Medicare HMOs instead. (See Chapter 8 for a discussion of Medicare HMOs.)

The Extension of Medicare to the Disabled and to Those with Kidney Failure

Within a few years of the enactment of Medicare, Congress made some additions to the program that were to have significant long-term policy impacts. The first was to extend eligibility for the program to disabled persons under 65. People who are determined to be permanently disabled are eligible to receive Social Security benefits before they turn 65. As part of this benefit, in 1972 they were also included in Medicare.

Before the 1960s, there was no effective treatment for people who developed kidney failure (referred to as end-stage renal disease, or ESRD). Those who got ESRD usually died. During the 1960s the technology of kidney dialysis was developed. As with most new technologies, dialysis was very expensive and was in short supply. It became apparent that this lifesaving alternative was available selectively to those with either the money or the insurance coverage to pay for it. Patients with ESRD who couldn't pay for it had no access to it and were left to die. This allocation of lifesaving technology according to the ability to pay was viewed with anathema by many in Congress. Such a policy was simply not consistent with American norms and values. Accordingly Congress acted to include all patients with ESRD in the Medicare program, regardless of age. The costs of dialysis would be paid by the government.

The decision to include ESRD under Medicare coverage was to have long–range effects that could not have been fully envisioned in 1972. The technology of surgical kidney transplantation was improving rapidly at this time. These costs were also paid by Medicare. The technology of dialysis has improved over the years, keeping more and more people alive, but also adding more and more to the cost of ESRD care. In the era of genetic engineering, new types of treatments were developed to improve the quality of life of ESRD patients. These newer treatments often cost as much as dialysis itself. Finally, in the era of the for-profit health care provider, the guaranteed availability of Medicare financing for all kidney care led to the development of a growing number of for-profit, investor-owned corporations providing kidney dialysis. A number of analysts have come to question the quality of the care provided by these for-profit dialysis centers, and the appropriateness of the federal government being the principal source of payment (and thus profit) for them. (See Chapter 7 for further discussion of these issues.)

In 1996, Medicare spent an average of $4996 per elderly beneficiary. The figure for beneficiaries eligible for Medicare due to ESRD was $24,835. The unexpected costs involved in fulfilling the federal commitment to equal access to lifesaving treatments to all with ESRD regardless of income has made Congress hesitant to invoke such egalitarian values again. With expensive, lifesaving treatments available for diseases such as acquired immune deficiency syndrome (AIDS), and with a growing number of poor individuals and families going without access to basic medical care, Congress has been unwilling to extend the values implied by the ESRD coverage to other diseases or groups.

The Rising Cost of Medicare

It didn't take long after the enactment of Medicare in 1965 for the costs of the program to become much larger than expected. Within a few years the cost of the program more than doubled, from $4.2 billion in 1967 to $9.3 billion in 1973. It doubled again between 1973 and 1977. As more and more people received Medicare coverage, and as the increasing availability of technology led to a rapidly rising cost of care, the cost of the program continued to balloon.

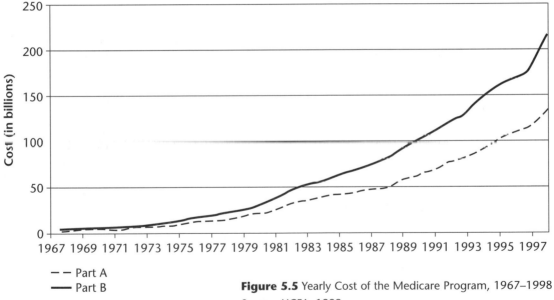

Figure 5.5 Yearly Cost of the Medicare Program, 1967–1998
Source: HCFA, 1999
Note: Costs are not adjusted for inflation.

Figure 5.5 shows the yearly cost of the Medicare program between 1967 and 1998. It shows the cost of Part B added to the cost of Part A to give the total cost for each year. By 1998 the cost of Medicare exceeded $200 billion, an increase of 50-fold over a period of 31 years. This amount is bigger than the national health budget of most other countries. It can also be seen from Figure 5.5 that the gap between Part A expenditures and Part B expenditures is increasing. More and more of the cost of Medicare is coming from Part B. Recall that 75% of the cost of Part B comes out of general tax revenues. This means that as Medicare continues to increase in cost over the next years and decades, an increasing strain will be placed on the federal budget.

In the 30 years since the original enactment of Medicare, Congress has made a number of policy changes in an attempt to hold down expenditures. The first of these came in 1972 with enactment of the system of professional standards review organizations, or PSROs. These were independent review bodies, often created as an offshoot of local medical societies, charged with reviewing the appropriateness of the hospital care provided to Medicare and Medicaid patients. It was thought that groups of community physicians could advise their peers on avoiding unnecessary hospital costs and thus reduce the cost of hospitalization. Though well intended, the PSROs had little effect on stemming the rise in hospital costs.

The next major step intended to reduce hospital costs was the prospective payment system (PPS), discussed in Chapter 3. Enacted in 1983, PPS reversed the incentives faced by hospitals, encouraging the rapid discharge of Medicare patients. The PPS was widely viewed as a success, with the increases in the cost of hospital care moderating substantially in the years following its enactment.

Changes in the Way Medicare Pays Physicians

As a result of the rising costs of Part B, Congress began to look closely at the fees it was paying physicians. The original schedule of acceptable fees for physician services was based on a weighted average of what other physicians in the same community charged for the same service, referred to as the usual, customary, and reasonable charge (UCR). The original Part B payment schedule would pay physicians 80% of UCR. Analysts within the federal Health Care Financing Administration and Congress began to question the level of the physicians' fees. Under directions from Congress, the government commissioned a detailed study of physicians' fees, and based on the results of these studies created the resource based relative value scale (RBRVS).

RBRVS created a system of measuring the actual resources that go into the provision of a medical service and assigning a value reflecting those resources, using a new scale based on the relative value unit (RVU). Every possible procedure was assigned a specific number of RVUs according to the resources required to perform the procedure. If one procedure involved twice as many RVUs as another, it was seen as requiring twice as many resources. Medicare simply established a standard payment rate per RVU, and used this figure to calculate the eligible charge for all procedures.

The Health Care Financing Administration (HCFA) is the federal agency that manages the Medicare program. Initially HCFA distinguished between an RVU involved in doing a procedure (e.g., surgery or repairing a broken bone) and an RVU involved in the ongoing evaluation and management of a patient (e.g., an office visit to treat high blood pressure). Physicians whose practice included procedures were paid more per RVU than those involved mainly in evaluation and management services. The debate continues as to whether procedural services and the services of evaluation and management should receive different levels of payment. HCFA has taken steps to equalize payment for the two services.

There have been two principal results of the shift to the RBRVS system of physician payment. One is that the historical income gap between surgeons and other procedure-oriented physicians on the one hand and primary care and other evaluation and management physicians on the other hand has narrowed substantially, due to increased payment for evaluation and management services and reduced payment for procedures.

Also, by creating a simplified fee schedule based on the concept of the RVU, it has become fairly straightforward for Congress and HCFA to control the amount paid to physicians. When the cost of physician care is seen as increasing too rapidly, HCFA has simply reduced the reimbursement per RVU, thus reducing payment to physicians overall.

Concept 5.5

The resource-based relative value scale (RBRVS) established a simplified method for paying physicians treating Medicare patients. Instituting the scale improved the equity in the way primary care physicians and procedural specialists are paid, and provided a mechanism for controlling overall Part B Medicare costs.

Even though the most rapid growth in Medicare has been in Part B, the most attention has been given to Part A. In the late 1990s government reports indicated that the Medicare Trust Fund (the fund that holds the money to pay for Part A services) was spending money faster than it was bringing it in, and if nothing were changed, the Trust Fund would go broke in 2001. These predictions started to come true. In 1997, for the first time, the Trust Fund spent more than it took in, by about $4 billion. As a result,

Congress passed a series of changes to Medicare as part of the Balanced Budget Act of 1997. These changes in the Medicare program and their effects are discussed in Chapter 8.

Taking Care of the Few: The Skewed Nature of the Medicare Population

Increases in life expectancy for all Americans and changes in demographic patterns are having a substantial impact on the cost of Medicare. When Medicare was established in the 1960s approximately 9.5% of the population of the country was 65 years or older. A man who was 65 years old at that time could expect to live an additional 13 years on average (17 for a woman). By 1990 12.3% of the population was 65 or older, and additional life expectancy at age 65 had increased to 15.1 years for men and 18.9 years for women. Current HCFA projections indicate that this proportion of the population 65 or over will rise to 12.9% by 2010 and 19.9% by 2030.

Of the Medicare population, the sector that is increasing the fastest is those over 85 years of age. These "frail elderly" have many more chronic medical problems and use many more medical resources than younger Medicare beneficiaries. In 1996, Medicare spent on average $4996 per elderly beneficiary. However, this amount varies widely depending on the health of the beneficiary. For example, in 1996 the average annual expenditure for beneficiaries who rate their health as "poor" is $11,739, while the figure for those who rate their health as "excellent" is $2134.

Figure 5.6 shows the distribution of 1996 Medicare spending for elderly beneficiaries. The solid bars indicate what percentage of total Medicare spending is accounted for by beneficiaries whose medical care costs are above the indicated level. Thus it can be seen that 5% of Medicare beneficiaries had annual expenditures of more than $25,000, accounting for 45% of all spending. By contrast, the healthiest 52% of beneficiaries had annual expenditures of less than $1000 and accounted for only 3% of total spending. Less than half of the elderly Medicare population accounts for 97% of all spending; 14% of the population accounts for 73% of spending.

Concept 5.6

Medicare spends most of its money taking care of a very few people: the care of 23% of the elderly population uses 85% of Medicare funds.

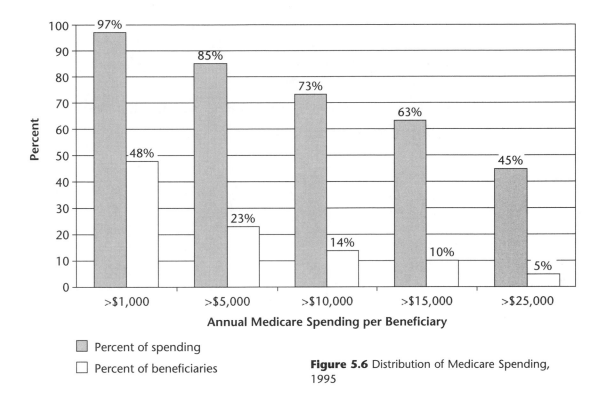

Figure 5.6 Distribution of Medicare Spending, 1995

Two additional points should be made about the Medicare program. As discussed above, the cost of providing medical care to the elderly has become increasingly expensive over time. The result has been that most current beneficiaries receive substantially more in benefits—in the range of to 5–10 times more—than they contributed to the system during their working years. Medicare is a system based on shifting financial resources from current workers to current elderly.

The second point has to do with the administrative efficiency of the Medicare system. During the debate over national health care reform in 1993–1994, opponents made much of the added federal bureaucracy that would be developed if the Clinton reform proposals were adopted. The implication was that giving the government greater responsibility in administering health care resources would lead to massive inefficiency.

The Medicare system, despite being one of the largest government programs in history, has proven to be one of the most efficient administrative systems for providing health care to a defined population of patients. A common measure of efficiency in health care is the percentage of all costs that goes to administration rather than patient care. Employer-based insurance typically spends 10–30% of costs on administration and other expenses unrelated to patient care (e.g., corporate profit). For nonprofit HMOs such as Kaiser-Permanente this figure is in the range of 3–7%. In 1996, Medicare Part A spent 1.0% of all funds on administrative costs; the figure for Part B was 2.6%.

> ## Concept 5.7
>
> The administrative structure of Medicare, managed by the federal Health Care Financing Administration, is the most efficient medical payment system in the country.

Strange Bedfellows: Medicare and Paying for Graduate Medical Education

Graduate medical education (GME) refers to the training physicians receive after they graduate from medical school. It includes training offered in residency programs and specialty fellowship programs. Since 1983 the federal government has taken principal responsibility for paying the costs of GME, essentially reimbursing most of the cost of the training to hospitals that offer GME. For reasons explained below, the cost of GME is paid out of the Medicare Part A Trust Fund. For decades no limits were placed on the number of GME positions that could be funded, resulting in a powerful financial incentive for hospitals to increase the size of their GME programs. The result was a dramatic increase in the number of available GME slots and an influx of doctors graduating from foreign medical schools (referred to as foreign medical graduates, or FMGs) in order to fill those slots. Of all the doctors in GME training programs in the United States today, approximately one in four is an FMG.

In the 1990s the cost to the government for this program increased until it accounted for approximately 7% of all Part A spending. It may seem odd that the program intended to pay for hospital care for seniors has taken on responsibility for paying the costs of GME. Such a perception is accurate, and represents a strange and unintended twist in the history of Medicare.

As described in Chapter 3, Medicare was not initially intended to be the principal source of funding for GME. However, as a result of a political compromise enacted at the time the prospective payment system was initiated in 1983, Medicare became responsible for paying most of the costs of GME. The system worked relatively well for a number of years. It became readily apparent to hospitals that by increasing the number of GME slots, they would increase the subsidy they would receive from the federal government. For many hospitals, particularly inner-city hospitals that provide care to low-income patients, resident physicians provide the bulk of the care (albeit under the supervision of fully trained physicians on the hospital staff). The Medicare payments for GME provided a source of inexpensive humanpower for these hospitals. These and other hospitals throughout the country responded by increasing their GME slots. The effect on the system overall was a growing surplus of GME training slots when compared to the number of medical students graduating from United States medical schools. It became necessary for hospitals to look to FMG physicians to fill their training programs, with a resulting influx of FMG physicians into the country. A substantial majority of FMG physicians trained in the United States under this program remain in the country after their training is completed. Thus the federal government, despite never intending to do so, created and for years maintained a program that put a substantial drain on the Medicare Part A Trust Fund and added to the growing surplus of physicians (particularly specialists) in the country.

Major Policy Questions Facing Medicare

As we move into the twenty-first century, and as a growing segment of the population is eligible for Medicare, the federal government will face a number of serious policy questions regarding the future of Medicare. As discussed in Chapter 8, Congress and HCFA have taken a number of steps in recent years intended to strengthen Medicare. Few would argue that these steps have solved Medicare's ongoing problems. Maintaining the long-term stability of the Medicare program will continue to be a major challenge to physicians, policy makers, and the public for years to come. Some of the questions that need to be addressed are outlined below.

How Should the Trust Fund Be Made Financially Sound?

There continue to be questions about the long-term stability of the Part A Trust Fund. Before the baby-boom generation comes fully into retirement age, we will have to decide how to maintain the fund's financial stability. The choices include the following:

- Increase payroll taxes
- Decrease payment rates to hospitals
- Increase the amount patients pay for care
- Limit the care available

- Encourage patients to enroll in HMOs
- Require patients to enroll in HMOs

How Should Rising Part B Costs Be Covered?

Seventy-five percent of the funding for Part B comes from the general federal treasury. After years of running huge budget deficits, the federal government currently is enjoying a substantial budget surplus. As Part B costs escalate, choices for paying them include the following:

- Continue to pay for Part B out of the surplus
- Increase patients' premiums
- Increase patients' share of the cost in addition to premiums (i.e., deductibles, copayments)
- Decrease payment to doctors
- Institute a sliding scale of premiums for Medicare patients
- Encourage (require) patients to join an HMO
- Initiate a capitation payment mechanism for Part B, similar to the prospective payment mechanism for Part A

Should the Separation of Part A and Part B Be Maintained?

It is important to recall that the original decision to split Medicare into two parts reflected a political compromise rather than a consensus about optimal system design. With the growing role of integrated health systems such as HMOs, many suggest that Medicare should be rebuilt from the ground up, with one integrated program of services and one comprehensive, stable financing mechanism. A change of this magnitude would also allow Medicare to incorporate a medigap option into its program, a proposal many policy analysts support.

Will Attempts at Cost Savings by Reducing Fees to Physicians and Hospitals Result in Decreased Access to Care?

Doctors and hospitals are not required to see Medicare patients. If Medicare further reduces the level of its payments to doctors (already lower than many private insurance plans) and hospitals, will these providers simply stop seeing Medicare patients? If so, where will Medicare patients get care?

ON-LINE DATA SOURCES

The data used in this chapter come from the United States Health Care Financing Agency (HCFA), the agency within the Department of Health and Human Services charged with administering the Medicare program. Extensive information about Medicare and other federal programs is available at www.hcfa.gov/.

Compilations of statistics about Medicare are available at
  www.hcfa.gov/stats/stats.htm. Many of these files can be downloaded
  as a pdf file. Two of the most helpful are the Medicare Chart Book
  and the annual compilation of national health care data.
Actuarial estimates about future aspects of Medicare are available at
  www.hcfa.gov/pubforms/tr/hi1999/hi6.htm.
Detailed information about the RBRVS is available at
  www.hcfa.gov/medicare/wrvu%2Dch1.htm.

REFERENCES

Ball RM. What Medicare's Architects Had in Mind. *Health Affairs* 1995;
  14(4):62–72. (A description of the origins of Medicare and the political
  maneuvering surrounding its enactment.)

CHAPTER 6

Medicaid

Key Concepts

- Medicaid differs from Medicare in three important ways:

  Rather than being universally available to all poor people, it covers only certain subgroups.

  Rather than combining a service plan and an insurance plan, it is strictly an insurance plan.

  Rather than being administered by the federal government, it is administered by the states under broad federal guidelines.

- Under the Medicaid program, eligi-

  bility for benefits, the level of benefits, and the average cost of car vary widely among states.

- Seventy-four percent of Medicaid costs go to provide care for 30% of beneficiaries: the low-income elderly and disabled, many of whom are in nursing homes. Low-income families and children account for about 25% of Medicaid costs.

- Over the period of 1991–1999, Med icaid shifted from a predominantly fee-for-service system to a system based predominantly on capitation and the use of HMOs.

In 1965 the U.S. Congress made sweeping changes in the way health care is financed and provided. It established Medicare, the program to provide health care to the elderly, discussed in the previous chapter. At the same time Congress enacted Medicaid, a program to provide health care to the poor. Like Medicare, Medicaid was created as an amendment to the existing Social Security Act, and thus is often referred to as Title XIX.

Unlike Medicare, which covers all elderly people in the country who qualify for Social Security, Medicaid is not a program for all people who fall below the poverty line. It pays for care only for certain subgroups of the poor. Also in contrast to Medicare, Medicaid is structured purely on an insurance model, with no direct service component. Finally, whereas Medicare is financed and administered purely by the federal government, Medicaid is administered by the states, with the federal government reimbursing each state for a portion of program costs.

Concept 6.1

Medicaid differs from Medicare in three important ways:

Rather than being universally available to all poor people, it covers only certain subgroups.

Rather than combining a service plan and an insurance plan, it is strictly an insurance plan.

Rather than being administered by the federal government, it is administered by the states under broad federal guidelines.

As with Medicare, the design and structure of the Medicaid program reflects historical and political factors that existed at the time of its passage. Prior to 1965, there was a federal program (the Kerr-Mills program) that distributed federal funds to each of the states to assist in paying for medical care for the elderly poor. This program had four principal characteristics:

1. It had a combination of federal and state funding.
2. It was administered by the states under broad federal guidelines.
3. Eligibility for the program was tied to eligibility for cash welfare grants.
4. So long as a state provided the basic benefits required by the federal government, it was free to set its own level of additional benefits.

When Congress enacted Medicaid, rather than actually going through the process of designing a new program, it simply replicated the characteristics of the Kerr Mills program. These four principles continue to define the structure of Medicaid today.

Under Medicaid, each state designs its own program for paying for medical care for the poor, using existing hospitals and doctors and initially paying for care on a fee-for-service basis. Its reliance on the existing system was seen as a way to bring the poor into the "mainstream" of American medical care. As discussed below, the rising costs of the program have made this goal very difficult to achieve.

Medicaid was established as a voluntary program for the states, with each state free to choose whether to participate. As a strong incentive, the federal government agreed to reimburse each participating state for a large part of the cost of the program. The actual share of the program that the federal government would pay depended on the economic condition of the state. States with lower per capita incomes have a higher share of the program costs paid by the federal government than do states with higher per capita incomes. For 2001, the federal share of the Medicaid program ranged from 50% in New York and Connecticut to 77% in Mississippi and 75% in West Virginia. In 1997 the federal government paid 56% of the overall cost of the Medicaid program.

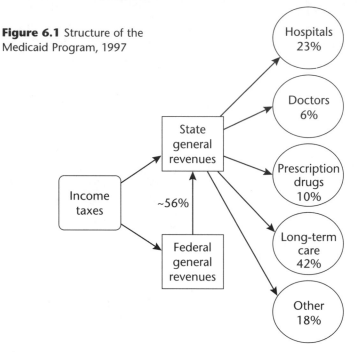

Figure 6.1 Structure of the Medicaid Program, 1997

As shown in Figure 6.1, the costs of the Medicaid program, whether state or federal, come straight out of general tax revenues. Thus on the pay stub shown in Figure 5.1, the employee is helping to pay for the program both through federal withholding tax and state withholding tax. As with Part B of Medicare, this reliance on general tax revenues means that at times of rapidly rising health care costs, a severe strain can be placed on both federal and state budgets. For this reason Medicaid costs continuously receive close scrutiny from lawmakers.

Services Provided Under the Medicaid Program

In order for a state Medicaid program to be eligible for reimbursement from the federal government, it must provide certain basic services to all enrollees. These include:

- Hospital care (inpatient and outpatient)
- Nursing home care

- Physician services
- Laboratory and X ray services
- Immunizations and other preventive services for children
- Family planning services
- Services provided at federally approved community health centers
- Nurse midwife and nurse practitioner services

In addition, states have the option of providing certain additional services for which they receive federal matching funds, including:

- Prescription drugs
- Institutional care for individuals with mental retardation
- Home- and community-based care for the frail elderly
- Personal care and other community-based services for individuals with disabilities
- Dental care and vision care

Figure 6.1 shows how the money in the Medicaid program is spent. Only 6% of all Medicaid funds goes to pay physicians, and 23% pays for hospital care. The cost of prescription drugs, one of the most rapidly rising parts of Medicaid costs, takes 10% of all funds. The largest share however, 42%, goes to pay for long-term care.

Eligibility for Medicaid

In order to be eligible for Medicaid, an individual must be within one of the four groups listed next.

Members of Low-Income Families with Children

Historically, Medicaid eligibility for this group was tied to eligibility for cash welfare grants under the Aid to Families with Dependent Children (AFDC) program. However, the changes included in the welfare reform that was enacted in 1996 broke this link. Currently, families with children and with incomes that fall below the federal poverty line are eligible to receive Medicaid coverage. In addition, children under 6 who are in families that earn up to 133% of the poverty line are eligible for Medicaid (see Appendix 6.1). Pregnant women in families that earn up to 133% of the poverty line are also eligible for Medicaid coverage limited to paying for medical care during pregnancy and immediately after birth.

In 1997, Medicaid covered approximately 21 million low-income children and 8.6 million low-income adults in families with children. Most of the eligible adults were women. This represents a decline in coverage of approximately 1.6 million since 1995, the year before welfare reform took effect (Kaiser Family Foundation 1999).

Elderly Who Meet Certain Income Requirements

People over 65 whose income is below a level established by the federal government qualify for supplemental cash payments under the Supplemental Security Income (SSI) program. People eligible for SSI are also eligible for Medicaid. In 1997 approximately 1.8 million people were eligible in this manner.

A second group of the elderly have income that is higher than the allowable Medicaid limits but face medical expenses that are more than they can pay. Before these people become eligible for Medicaid they must first use most of their personal savings to pay for their medical care. After they "spend down" their savings to a certain level (usually a few thousand dollars), they become eligible for Medicaid. Most people eligible for Medicaid in this manner are confined to a nursing home. In 1997 approximately 2 million additional elderly were eligible for Medicaid in this manner.

As discussed in Chapter 9, Medicare provides little in the way of coverage for nursing home care. Nonetheless a growing number of the elderly are facing the prospect of nursing home care without the means to pay for it. They turn to the Medicaid program as the payer of last resort.

Disabled Persons

People with long-term disabilities qualify for Medicaid in the same manner as the elderly. Disabled people who receive cash payments from SSI are also eligible for Medicaid. In addition, disabled persons not covered by SSI but incurring large medical expenses are eligible for Medicaid after they meet the spend-down requirements. In 1997 approximately 6.8 million individuals with disabilities were covered by Medicaid. As with the elderly, many of these individuals are confined to hospitals, nursing homes, or other institutional care facilities on a long-term basis.

There are certain other general requirements that all Medicaid beneficiaries must meet, including in most cases American citizenship. Certain legal immigrants are eligible depending on their date of entry into the country. Those immigrants who entered the country illegally are ineligible for Medicaid except for emergency care. If a woman who has entered the country illegally has a baby at a hospital in the United States, the baby is automatically a U.S. citizen, and thus eligible for Medicaid (assuming the family meets the income requirements), but the mother remains ineligible.

Other Groups

In order for a state to qualify for federal reimbursement, all members of the preceding three groups within a state must be eligible for Medicaid. In addition, states have the option of receiving federal reimbursement for covering other groups, including

1. Pregnant women and infants under the age of one whose family earns up to 185% of the poverty line
2. Elderly, blind, or disabled persons who are not eligible for SSI payments but still have incomes below the federal poverty line
3. Children up to the age of 21 in certain low-income families

Finally, each state has the option of covering individuals who are not in one of the above groups but whose income falls below a level set by the state. These are the "medically needy." Most of these are low-income single adults or families without children. Because each state establishes its own cutoff level for eligibility, and because general economic conditions vary substantially from state to state, there is a wide range of eligibility levels among the states. Few states cover all poor people in this category. Most states have established income eligibility levels that are a fraction of the federal poverty level, often as low as 30–40%.

In 1997 Medicaid spent an average of $3862 per beneficiary. Because the program is administered by the states, which have a wide range of options in eligibility and coverage, the average level of Medicaid spending per eligible beneficiary varies widely among states. In 1997 spending per beneficiary ranged from $2397 in Tennessee and $2543 in California to $7373 in Connecticut and $7595 in New York.

Poor people who are eligible for care in one state are often ineligible in another. Treatments covered in one state may not be covered in another. The wide latitude left to states in creating their Medicaid programs and the resulting wide range of eligibility and coverage among the states has created a system of medical care for the poor that is distinctly different from our system of care for the elderly. Medicare is essentially government-sponsored, taxpayer-supported, universal care for the elderly. Medicaid is a program intended to cover certain segments of the low-income population and leaves other segments without the means to pay for medical care. As John Iglehart has stated,

> *The nature of the Medicaid program underscores the ambivalence of a society that has never decided which of its citizens deserves access to publicly financed medical care or whether the problem of poverty should be addressed primarily at the national, state, or local level. . . . This situation constitutes what has been characterized as "the greatest inequity of the American health care system . . .*

not between the nonpoor and the poor, but between the insured poor and the uninsured poor." (Iglehart 1993, p. 896)

Concept 6.2

Under the Medicaid program, eligibility for benefits, the level of benefits, and the average cost of care vary widely among states.

The Rising Costs of the Medicaid Program

Between 1975 and 1997 the overall cost of the Medicaid program grew from $12 billion to more than $160 billion. Even after adjusting for inflation, this represents a tripling of program expenditures during this period.

Between 1975 and 1989 the cost of the program increased by an average of 11.9% per year before adjusting for inflation. Reflecting both the rising cost of care nationwide and the increasing eligibility for program coverage, in 1989 program costs began to explode. Between 1989 and 1993 the yearly increase in overall Medicaid costs averaged 21.2%. As a result of these increases both the federal government (which was already facing huge budget deficits as a result of changes in the tax laws enacted in the 1980s) and state governments (many of which were prevented by their state constitutions from engaging in deficit spending) were facing financial crises. If nothing were done to change the program, Medicaid threatened to bankrupt many of the states and the federal government. As discussed below, the federal government responded by initiating a number of changes on a state-by-state basis. Medicaid rapidly began to change from a purely fee-for-service payment system to a system of capitation, shifting much of the financial risk of providing care to the poor from governments to HMOs and other types of insurers and providers.

A common misperception at that time was that, since Medicaid is primarily a program for low-income families and children, the rapid increase in program costs was due to an explosion of the welfare rolls and an increasing problem with welfare fraud and abuse. This picture is not at all accurate, and constitutes one of the major public misperceptions regarding our health care system.

It is true that low-income children and adults make up nearly 66% of Medicaid beneficiaries. However, as shown in Figure 6.2, these groups combined account for about 25% of overall Medicaid spending. The bulk of Medicaid expenditures (74% in 1997) pay for care for low-income elderly and disabled individuals.

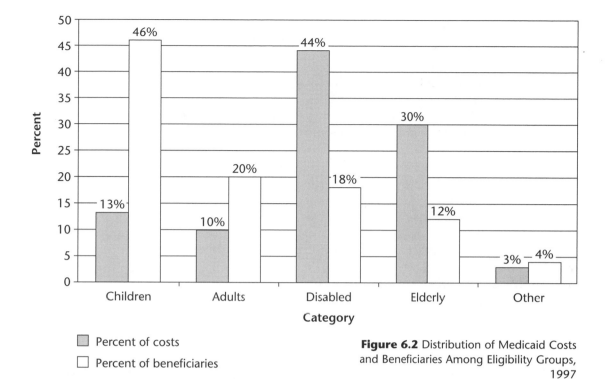

Percent of costs
Percent of beneficiaries

Figure 6.2 Distribution of Medicaid Costs and Beneficiaries Among Eligibility Groups, 1997

Concept 6.3

Seventy-four percent of Medicaid costs go to provide care for 30% of beneficiaries: the low-income elderly and disabled, many of whom are in nursing homes. Low-income families and children account for about 25% of Medicaid costs.

If one looks at the average cost of providing care for beneficiaries in each class of eligibility, shown in Table 6.1, it is easy to see how this situation arises. Medicaid has come to be our society's safety net that ensures that no elderly or disabled individual who needs care in a nursing home or other long-term care institution will be left without care due to inability to pay.

There also is a common misperception that Medicaid beneficiaries abuse the medical care system and overuse medical services. Critics frequently cite data about the high rate at which Medicaid patients use hospital emergency rooms to obtain routine medical care. It is very expensive to take care of common, nonemergency conditions in the emergency room.

In many areas it is true that Medicaid beneficiaries are more likely than the general public to use the emergency room rather than doctors' offices

Table 6.1

Medicaid Expenditures per Beneficiary, 1997

Type of Beneficiary	Average Annual Expenditure
Elderly	$9540
Disabled	$8832
Children	$1026
Adults	$1809

Source: HCFA

for the treatment of relatively minor ailments. The reason does not appear to be abusive behavior on the part of Medicaid patients but rather the poor availability of primary care services for those on Medicaid.

Soon after its creation in 1965 most states began to restrict the amount they would pay physicians for treating Medicaid patients. As Medicaid costs skyrocketed in the 1980s and 1990s, states cut back even further on what they were willing to pay. Doctors in many areas of the country now receive only 30–40% of their usual charge for taking care of a Medicaid patient. As a result of these payment policies,

Approximately one-third of doctors won't treat any Medicaid patients.

Approximately one-third of doctors will treat their established patients on Medicaid but won't take new patients.

Approximately one-third of doctors will treat Medicaid patients who are new to their practice.

This poor availability of doctors is largely responsible for the general relationship illustrated in Figure 6.3 between the rate at which Medicaid patients use office-based primary care services in a community and the rate

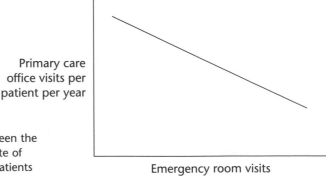

Figure 6.3 General Relationship Between the Availability of Primary Care and the Rate of Emergency Room Visits for Medicaid Patients

Source: De Alteris and Fanning 1991

at which they visit the emergency room. The more available office-based or clinic-based primary care services are to Medicaid patients, the less those patients visit the emergency room. Making primary care more available to Medicaid recipients will help to decrease emergency room utilization and will lower the overall cost of care somewhat. However, as we see in Chapter 11, other factors besides insurance coverage impair the availability of primary care to low-income families and individuals.

The Move to Managed Care

In the face of rapidly rising costs, both state and federal governments began to look for ways to limit the budgetary drain of Medicaid. By the early 1990s HMOs and the other types of managed care plans discussed in Chapter 4 were increasingly common in many areas of the country. It was apparent to federal and state officials that delivery systems based on the capitation method of payment had the potential of realizing the same cost savings for Medicaid patients as they did for patients in general. With the support of the federal government, many states established programs to enroll as many Medicaid beneficiaries as possible in HMOs. (In most states elderly or disabled Medicaid beneficiaries were not included in the shift to HMOs.) The state would pay a fixed premium per patient per year, and it would be up to the HMO to constrain costs.

Figure 6.4 shows the rapid movement of Medicaid from a system based predominantly on fee-for-service payment to doctors and hospitals to one that had more than half of its beneficiaries in managed care plans in 1999.

Concept 6.4

Over the period of 1991-1999, Medicaid shifted from a predominantly fee-for-service system to a system based predominantly on capitation and the use of HMOs.

In order for states to move their Medicaid beneficiaries from the fee-for-service system into HMOs and other managed care plans, a mechanism had to be developed to relax the federal guidelines that states must meet to qualify for federal reimbursement. The original guidelines required states to provide all necessary services in the categories described above. As discussed in Chapter 4, HMOs save money by putting certain constraints on the use of hospitals and other expensive technologies. In order to reconcile the guidelines with the need to shift patients into HMOs, Congress amended Section 1115 of the Social Security Act to allow the secretary of

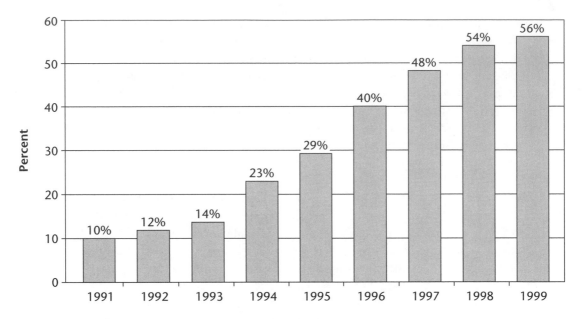

Figure 6.4 Percentage of Medicaid Enrollees in Managed Care, 1991–1999
Source: HCFA

the Department of Health and Human Services to waive certain guidelines on a state-by-state basis. States could apply for a "Section 1115 waiver" to create capitated systems of care for certain of their Medicaid beneficiaries. These waivers are granted for periods of five years at a time, and are renewable for additional periods of five years. They allow states to enter into contracts with HMOs or other managed care organizations to provide care for Medicaid beneficiaries. Under the contract the HMO receives a regular capitation payment from the state for each member enrolled and assumes full risk for the costs of providing care to these members. These contracts are thus referred to as "risk contracts."

By 1999, 17 states had completed Section 1115 waivers, accounting for the increase in managed care enrollment shown in Figure 6.4. Some of these waiver programs worked quite well, but others had serious problems. Some were quite controversial. In the following section we look at the experience of three states in creating managed care programs under these 1115 waivers.

The Oregon Plan: Explicit Health Care Rationing

In the late 1980s Oregon was facing the same run-up in Medicaid costs that other states were confronting. The cost of the Medicaid program had put such a strain on the state budget that Oregon was able to pay for care for only a fraction of its poor population. Medicaid was available only to those with an income less than about 60% of the poverty line, leaving those with incomes between 60% and 100% of the poverty line without any coverage at all. Oregon wanted to find a way to provide care for all people below the poverty line and for pregnant women and children whose family income was less than 133% of the poverty line. They wanted to do this, however, without increasing the overall amount they spent on Medicaid.

In order to accomplish these seemingly irreconcilable goals, the Oregon legislature, under the leadership of one of its members who was also a physician, created an entirely new way of allocating Medicaid resources. This new program, referred to as the Oregon Health Plan (OHP), took an entirely new approach to the allocation of Medicaid funds. A broadly representative commission called the Oregon Health Services Commission underwent a lengthy process of studying all the services previously covered by Medicaid and dividing them into approximately 700 treatment categories. The commission then ranked these treatments based on factors such as medical effectiveness, ability to avert death or disability, prevention of future costs, and public health risk. Treatments that ranked highest on these criteria (for example, treatment of severe head injuries or insulin-dependent diabetes) were given low numbers and those that ranked lowest (for example treatment of viral colds and simple strains of back muscles) were given high numbers. The Oregon Health Commission spent three years establishing this list. They had many public meetings and discussions of the plan, and modified earlier versions of the plan based on this input.

Figure 6.5 illustrates the situation that existed before the OHP was established. The horizontal axis shows the 700 treatment categories, ranked from most important to least important. The vertical axis shows the poor population of Oregon, ranked according to the percentage of the poverty line represented by their family income. Before the OHP, there was a sharp dividing line at about 60% of the poverty line, with those below the line receiving full Medicaid coverage for all 700 services and those above the line receiving no coverage at all.

In establishing the OHP, the Oregon legislature decided to remove some of the least effective treatments from coverage. It used the money saved by limiting care in this way to provide coverage for the most effective treatments for everyone below the poverty line, and for pregnant women and children below 133% of the poverty line. These changes are represented in Figure 6.6.

As shown in Figure 6.6, the OHP initially provided coverage for only 565 of the 700 available treatments, but it provided this limited coverage to all people below the poverty line. In order to reallocate its Medicaid funds in this way, Oregon first had to get a Section 1115 waiver from the federal

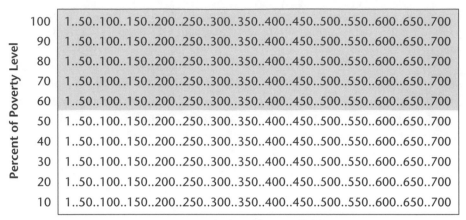

Figure 6.5 Medicaid Coverage in Oregon Before the Oregon Health Plan

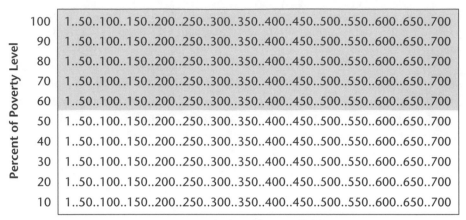

Figure 6.6 Medicaid Coverage Under the Oregon Health Plan

government. This waiver application was quite controversial. However, after several years of discussion and debate, the federal government approved the waiver, and in 1994 the Oregon Health Plan took effect. It has largely been successful in achieving its goal of increased coverage. In its first year of operation it extended coverage to approximately 100,000 more poor people in addition to the 188,000 originally covered. Although the plan has had a number of problems along the way, it continues to offer coverage to everyone in Oregon whose income is below the poverty line.

One of the ways the OHP tried to save money was to enroll as many of its members as possible in HMOs or other managed care plans and pay for their care under capitated risk contracts. It was quite successful in this effort, and by 1997 nearly 90% of beneficiaries were covered by a managed care plan.

The success of the OHP depended on broad public acceptance of the policy of limiting care to some so that others may be covered. Accusations of unethical health care rationing were leveled at the plan. This aspect of the plan and its implication for overall United States health care policy are discussed in Chapter 12.

Tennessee: Managed Care for All Medicaid Beneficiaries—Overnight

Tennessee faced a situation similar to that in Oregon: in the early 1990s costs were rising substantially, and coverage was limited to a fraction of Tennessee's poor population. Tennessee's previous Medicaid system was based almost exclusively on the traditional, fee-for-service model. Planners felt that if a substantial number of Medicaid beneficiaries were shifted from fee-for-service to capitated managed care, the money saved could be used to extend coverage not only to the entire poor population in Tennessee, but also to certain groups whose income was above the poverty line but who lacked health insurance. The problem in Tennessee was getting existing commercial HMOs and managed care plans to accept large numbers of Medicaid patients at capitation rates that were lower than prevailing market rates. Tennessee decided to use the power of the purse string to accomplish this. The legislature passed a law limiting the ability of health plans to enroll public school teachers and state employees to those plans that also agreed to accept Medicaid patients. Not wanting to lose access to one of the largest groups of employees in the state, most managed care plans in Tennessee agreed to accept Medicaid patients.

Tennessee applied to the federal government for a Section 1115 waiver to allow a shift from fee-for-service to managed care essentially overnight. On December 31, 1993, nearly all state Medicaid beneficiaries remained in the traditional fee-for-service system. On January 1, 1994, the new Tenncare program started, and virtually all Medicaid patients became members of a managed care plan.

The rapidity of the shift to managed care created an initial period of confusion and frustration for many patients and providers. Typical of most managed care plans, Medicaid patients were limited to receiving care from the specific plan in which they were enrolled. The problem was that many patients did not understand the way managed care was intended to work. Medicaid beneficiaries had been given a short time in which to select a managed care provider. Those who did not select a plan from the dozen or so plans on the list were assigned at random to one plan. In many cases patients were assigned to plans that did not include their regular provider of care. Other patients who did select a plan did so without a complete list of providers or a full understanding of the limits of managed care. For months, patients would show up at their usual provider, only to be told that they were ineligible for care. Often the provider they had been assigned to was a substantial distance away. Many providers were also frustrated at being unable to continue to provide care to patients they had known for years.

Over time the initial confusion subsided, and Tenncare achieved many of its objectives. In 1994, its first year of operation, Tenncare extended eligibility to 350,000 people over and above the 770,000 people previously in Medicaid. Over time, though, it has developed a number of serious problems. The cost of extending coverage to people with incomes over the poverty line who lacked health insurance turned out to be far more than expected. Many of these people lacked coverage for the very reason that they had chronic medical problems, and were thus "uninsurable." Tenncare has had to reduce its coverage to this group in order to save money. In addition, it has reduced the capitation rate it is willing to pay managed care providers who participate in the plan, leading some of the largest plans to withdraw from participation. Tenncare continues to be a model of the advantages and disadvantages of a rapid shift to managed care.

California: Incremental Shift to Medicaid Managed Care

The Medicaid program in California, referred to as Medi-Cal, is the nation's largest, with more than 5 million beneficiaries. In the 1980s California shared the experiences of most states with rapidly rising costs. Having previously extended program eligibility to many children in families with income above the poverty line, California shifted its policy focus to containing the cost of the Medi-Cal program. In order to do this, California obtained permission from the federal government to begin a statewide shift to managed care for most beneficiaries. As early as the 1970s California had enrolled certain Medi-Cal patients in HMOs. These early experiences had not been fully successful, so California adopted a somewhat cautious approach. Starting in the early 1990s California began to create managed care plans for Medi-Cal patients on a county-by-county basis. Each participating county had substantial flexibility in designing its plan. Three general types of plan were used:

1. A county-organized health system (COHS) to provide coverage on a capitated basis to all Medi-Cal patients within the county

2. A two-plan model, in which a COHS competed directly with a single commercial managed care plan
3. A market-based model, in which Medi-Cal beneficiaries within the county were free to choose from a list of competing, private managed care plans.

By early 1999, 2.3 million Medi-Cal patients, or 46% of the total enrollment, were enrolled in managed care plans statewide. The two-plan model was by far the most common, with 10 counties, including 1.7 million patients, choosing this approach. The remaining 600,000 patients were about evenly split between the two other options (Kaiser Family Foundation 2000).

Although the overall effectiveness of California's Medicaid reform, measured in terms of transferring beneficiaries to managed care plans, has been quite good, it has not been without its problems. Relying as it has on a county-by-county approach, the plan has proven to be complex from an administrative perspective. In addition, budgetary constraints in California have kept capitation payments to managed care providers quite low. Coupling low payments with what are perceived to be overly stringent program requirements, the plan has raised continuing questions about the quality of the care actually available to Medicaid recipients. However, the shift to managed care has made care more accessible. Patients who were having difficulty under the previous fee-for-service system due to low payment rates are now guaranteed access to a provider through their selected managed care plan.

The Long Term Outlook for Medicaid

As discussed above, Medicaid is moving toward becoming a system for providing care to poor people through managed care arrangements. Although the states differ, all of them benefit from a managed care structure for Medicaid, especially from the ability to control costs through capitated contracts, thus shifting the risk of cost escalation to the managed care providers.

It is unclear, however, just how successful this approach will be in containing overall Medicaid costs. Recall from Concept 6.3 that 74% of Medicaid costs go to provide care for 30% of beneficiaries: the low-income elderly and disabled, many of whom are in nursing homes. It is unclear to what extent the move to a managed care format for care will be able to contain the cost of providing care to these, the most vulnerable groups in our society. Recall from Chapter 4 that the effectiveness of capitated systems in reducing costs compared to fee-for-service systems is in reduced use of hospitals and other expensive technologies. It is not clear that paying the costs of caring for elderly and disabled poor people confined to nursing homes or other long-term care facilities can be reduced by capitation payment methods. In addition, the rapidly growing number of frail elderly people means that even more people will be turning to Medicaid to pay for their care. The bulk of the cost of Medicaid comes from the federal treasury. Despite a significant shift to managed care, the Medicaid system may well put continued strain on the federal budget for years to come.

ON-LINE DATA SOURCES

Data and analyses used in this chapter come from two principal sources: the Health Care Financing Administration within the United States Department of Health and Human Services, and a series of reports prepared by the Kaiser Family Foundation.

The Health Care Financing Administration has extensive information about Medicaid in the form of both narrative reports and data tables, available at www.hcfa.gov/medicaid/mcaidpti.htm.

In addition, HCFA publishes extensive data regarding Medicaid in its quarterly journal, *Health Care Financing Review*. Data for this chapter were taken from the 1999 statistical supplement to that journal.

The Kaiser Family Foundation is a nonprofit organization that works extensively on health policy issues. As part of its ongoing study of the Medicaid program it has prepared the following reports, all available on-line:

Medicaid: A Primer. 08/31/99, available at www.kff.org/content/1999/2161/pub2161.pdf.

Managed Care and Low-Income Populations: Four Years' Experience with the Oregon Health Plan. 08/31/99, available at www.kff.org/content/1999/2127/pub2127.pdf.

Managed Care and Low-Income Populations: Four Years' Experience with TennCare. 08/31/99, available at www.kff.org/content/1999/2129/pub2129.pdf.

Managed Care and Low-Income Populations: A Case Study of Managed Care in California. 04/30/00, available at www.kff.org/content/2000/2169/California-CaseStudy.pdf.

REFERENCES

De Alteris M, Fanning T. A Public Health Model of Emergency Room Use. *Health Care Financing Review*. 1991. 12(3):15–20.

Iglehart JK. The American Health Care System—Medicaid. *New England Journal of Medicine* 1993; 328:896–900.

APPENDIX 6.1

In this chapter we frequently refer to the federal poverty level, and where a family's income lies relative to that level. The following table shows this level for 1999, by size of family. Any family or individual that earned less than the amount shown was considered officially to be poor.

Federal Poverty Level by Size of Family for 1999

Size of Family Unit	Estimated Threshold of Poverty
1 person	$8,667
2 persons	11,214
3 persons	13,290
4 persons	17,028
5 persons	20,115
6 persons	22,719
7 persons	25,815
8 persons	28,788
9 persons or more	34,075

CHAPTER 7

The Managed Care Revolution

Key Concepts

- The growth in the number of HMOs in this country began in the years following the HMO Act of 1973. The changes the Reagan administration made to the HMO Act shifted HMOs from mostly nonprofit to predominantly for-profit.

- *Managed care* is a way of organizing and financing the direct delivery of care. *Managed competition* is a way of restructuring the entire health care system. It relies on managed care as the basic model for the delivery of care.

- Despite the failure of the U.S. Congress to enact national health care reform during the 1990s, market forces have acted to fundamentally restructure our system of health insurance. Most people in the United States with health insurance are now covered by some form of managed care plan.

- The move to managed care that took place in this country in the 1980s and 1990s appears to have realized a one-time savings in the amount we spend on health care, but appears to have failed to arrest the long-term growth in the overall cost of health care.

- Many of the reductions in care initiated by managed care companies in an effort to control costs have come to be perceived by the public as unwarranted reductions in quality.

- The widespread move to for-profit health care, and the need to maintain shareholder profits inherent in that move, have created additional pressures on the health care system to hold down costs. The expansion of for-profit care has compounded the public's negative reaction to managed care, creating the "managed care backlash."

A s discussed in Chapter 4, the development and expansion of the health maintenance organization (HMO) and other types of managed care delivery systems brought a fundamental change to health care in the United States. Driven largely by concerns over rising costs, the HMO Act of 1973 firmly established the role of the HMO in American health care. The federal government took a series of steps to promote the spread of

HMOs, including financial incentives and regulatory support. In order to be eligible for federal support, HMOs had to meet three basic requirements:

1. Offer a specified list of benefits to all members
2. Charge all members the same monthly premium, regardless of their health status (referred to as "community rating")
3. Be structured as a nonprofit organization

Ironically the initial effect of the HMO Act was the opposite of its intended effect: for an initial period it brought the creation of new HMOs in the United States to a grinding halt. The list of covered services required by the act was substantially more comprehensive than what was generally available in competing fee-for-service insurance plans. In order to provide the scope of benefits required by the government and to make these benefits available to all comers at the same price regardless of health status (something that competing fee-for-service plans definitely did *not* do), new HMOs would have been at a severe competitive disadvantage. As a consequence of these restrictions, no new HMOs were created in the two years following enactment of the plan.

Congress acted in 1976 to loosen the requirements HMOs must meet to receive federal financial and regulatory support, and the growth in HMOs began as intended. Within a year after the amendments to the act more than 50 new HMOs had qualified for federal support. By 1981, 10 million people were enrolled in HMOs nationwide. The growth of HMOs and similar plans has continued since that time, and in many areas of the country HMOs are now the rule rather than the exception (data on HMO enrollment from the Kaiser Family Foundation).

Initially the government maintained the requirement that qualifying HMOs be organized on a nonprofit basis. For the first several years of the expansion of HMOs, nearly the entire industry met this nonprofit requirement. In 1981 nearly 90% of HMO patients were members of nonprofit plans. However, the 1980s brought a fundamental change to the American political landscape. Ronald Reagan was elected president and a Republican majority was elected to the Senate. Fundamental to President Reagan's free-market philosophy, legislation was introduced to end the government's ability to regulate HMOs. By 1988, the end of President Reagan's term in office, Congress had eliminated all federal funding for new HMOs and had relaxed considerably the criteria that HMOs had to meet to obtain federal certification. If HMOs were to survive and prosper in the market for health insurance, they would have to do so on their own.

Chapter 4 also describes the American Medical Association's resistance throughout much of the twentieth century to HMOs and other delivery mechanisms based on the capitation method of payment. Looking at the history of HMOs in the years following the HMO Act and its modification by President Reagan, it is clear that once HMOs were out of the box they could never be put back. Between 1981 and 1989 enrollment in HMOs more than tripled, with more than 30 million people enrolled.

An additional change made during the Reagan years was to have a profound effect on the structure of health care in America. Congress removed the requirement that federally certified HMOs function on a nonprofit basis. As a harbinger of things to come, by 1989 nearly half of all HMOs operated on a for-profit basis.

Concept 7.1

The growth in the number of HMOs in this country began in the years following the HMO Act of 1973. The changes the Reagan administration made to the HMO Act shifted HMOs from mostly nonprofit to predominantly for-profit.

The growth in HMOs continued throughout the 1990s. By 1998, 79 million people were enrolled in HMOs. Nearly two-thirds of this enrollment was in for-profit plans. Over a period of 25 years the United States had shifted from a health care system organized almost exclusively on a fee-for-service basis to one organized around HMOs and other forms of capitated, managed care delivery. In addition, the provision of health insurance has changed from a largely nonprofit industry to one in which for-profit corporations predominate. At the center of this change has been a new concept: managed competition. Managed competition has redefined the way employers, health insurers, health care providers, and patients relate to each other.

Managed Competition: An Idea Whose Time Had Come

At certain times in a nation's political history, windows of opportunity open, allowing for the possibility of major social and political change. As described by John Kingdon (1984), three conditions must coexist in order for major policy changes to take place:

1. A policy issue must rise to the top of the national agenda, with broad public awareness and support.

2. The political circumstances prevailing at the time must be amenable to significant change in policy.

3. A plan for change must be available that offers realistic solutions to the problems that are present.

In the period 1992–1994, many people thought a window of opportunity had opened for major reform of our national health care system. The election of President Clinton put the need for health care reform close to the top of the national policy agenda. Members of Congress appeared broadly to support the need for change. A plan was immediately available that offered a compelling theoretical model of the new form health care in America could take: managed competition.

In 1980, in the midst of the changes to the health care industry described above, Alain Enthoven of Stanford University published a book entitled *Health Plan: The Only Practical Solution to the Soaring Cost of Medical Care.* This book proposed a national system of health care centered on the concept of groups of health care purchasers banding together to obtain health insurance from competing health insurers.

Under general economic theory, markets will function efficiently only when well-informed consumers are able to choose from among competing products. Both the producer and the consumer of a good or service should approach a potential market transaction on an equal basis. However, a purely market approach to providing health insurance or health care involves a number of inherent problems regarding this classical economic theory. (See Arrow 1963 for a more complete discussion of these issues.) Potential problems include inequality in the information available to physician and patient, the likelihood that merely having health insurance will increase the rate at which people access health care services (referred to as the "moral hazard" of health insurance), and the uncertainty involved in predicting the rate at which health services will be provided in the future.

Addressing these problems, Enthoven developed a proposal to reform the market for health insurance and health care to make it more efficient. He predicted that if the market were modified through regulation in order to counteract the forces that create market failure, "the health care system would be transformed, gradually and voluntarily, from today's system with built-in cost-increasing incentives to a system with built-in incentives for consumer satisfaction and cost control." He proposed "a system of fair economic competition in which consumers and providers of care, making decisions in an appropriately structured private market, would do the work of reorganization" (Enthoven 1980, pp. xxi–xxii). Building on this original work, in 1989 Enthoven collaborated with Richard Kronick to propose a modification of this original plan, called the "consumer choice health plan" (Enthoven and Kronick, 1989) The ideas contained in these plans form the core of proposals for national health care reform based on the concept of managed competition.

A major tenet of Enthoven's proposals for managed competition is that, by relying on market forces the country can address problems of rising costs to improve efficiency. By removing many of the constraints that have led to past market failures, managed competition would encourage the spread of health care organizations and delivery systems that are able to reduce unnecessary expenditures while maintaining quality.

Managed competition relies on four basic principles for the organization of the health care system:

1. Rather than selecting and purchasing health insurance directly through their employer, employees from a variety of companies would join together to form a "health insurance purchasing cooperative," often referred to as a HIPC (pronounced "hip'-pick").

2. These HIPCs would in turn shop among HMOs and other managed health care plans to select the best options for their members. The HIPCs would be large enough to have professional staff able to evaluate the quality of the care offered by the various plans available. On the basis of this quality assessment the HIPCs would select several plans to offer to members, thus ensuring a range of choice for members. The HIPCs would offer only plans that in the opinion of HIPC managers offered high quality at competitive prices.

3. All managed care plans that wanted to compete for the business of the HIPC would be required to offer a basic benefit package, covering a specified range of health care services. Historically it has been difficult for consumers to compare the price of competing health insurance plans, because each plan would have its own unique set of covered services. By ensuring that the benefit package was the same for all plans offered, consumers could make a direct price comparison of plans.

4. HMOs and other health plans competing for the business of the HIPCS would be free to offer coverage options that were more comprehensive than the basic benefit package. However, if a consumer selected a more comprehensive (and thus more expensive) option, the consumer would have to pay the added cost (that is, the difference between the plan selected and the basic plan) out of his or her own pocket. This added cost of the comprehensive plan would not be tax deductible, thus requiring the consumer to pay the full additional amount. (Recall from Concept 4.2 that current tax laws encourage consumers to buy more health insurance than they would buy if they were paying for it themselves. This aspect of managed competition would require the federal government to change the tax laws.)

Under managed competition, all privately purchased health insurance would be obtained through HIPCs. HIPCs would be organized on a regional basis, with one HIPC per region. The exception to this would be that employers with more than 1000 employees could act as their own HIPC. Any type of health plan, from a staff model HMO through a purely fee-for service PPO, would be permitted to offer coverage through the HIPC. However, a health plan that did not meet the standard of quality established by the HIPC would not be offered as an option to HIPC members. An exclusion of this type could mean the demise of noncompetitive plans. The theory of managed competition is illustrated in Figure 7.1.

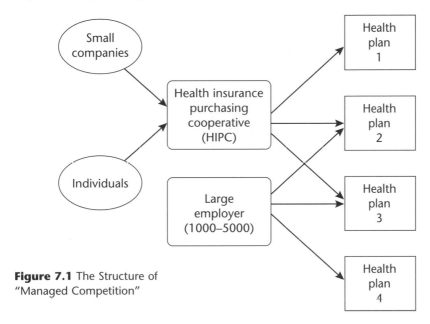

Figure 7.1 The Structure of "Managed Competition"

At this point it is important to clarify the difference between two fundamental concepts: managed care and managed competition.

Managed care is a means of organizing, paying for, and providing health care directly to consumers. It is paid for through a capitation arrangement, under which a particular group or organization is responsible for ensuring that all necessary care is provided to a given population of patients, and that the cost of that care does not exceed budgeted funds available. (The budget would be equal to the capitation rate times the number of members.) The responsible group then "manages" the care process to ensure that the budget is not exceeded. The responsible group may be

- An insurance company
- A nonprofit corporation
- A for-profit corporation
- Physicians and hospitals in combination

Managed competition, by contrast, is a system for providing health care on a regional basis, in which patients choose between competing systems of managed care.

Managed care is a way of providing care directly to consumers. Managed competition is a theory of health care reform that relies on managed care as the basis of health care organizing, financing, and delivery.

Concept 7.2

Managed care is a way of organizing and financing the direct delivery of care.

Managed competition is a way of restructuring the entire health care system. It relies on managed care as the basic model for the delivery of care.

Initially, critics of managed competition pointed out that the model was only a theoretical one that had never been tested. Even Enthoven and Kronick acknowledged that "the only proved method for bringing the growth in total expenditures into line with the gross national product is for government to take over most of health care financing and place it under firm global budgets." However, they concluded that "in view of our historic preferences for limited government and decentralization," it would be more effective in the case of the United States to create a private, market-based system of managed competition that is based on "generally accepted economic theory" (Enthoven and Kronick 1989, pp. 100–101).

According to Enthoven's view of economic theory, a properly organized market will, over time, lead to the efficient provision of health care. "Efficient" in this case refers to providing cost-effective care. As discussed in Chapter 2, a common measure of economic efficiency compares the relationship between marginal benefits and marginal costs. If the marginal benefits of an activity equal or exceed the marginal cost of acquiring those added benefits, it makes economic sense to take on the added cost. If marginal benefits turn out to be less than their marginal cost, it makes little sense to make the added investment. Efficiency is achieved at that point at which marginal benefits and marginal costs are approximately equal.

Applying this concept to health care, efficiency is achieved when the marginal benefits of additional care approximate the marginal cost, either for a specific health plan or for the system as a whole. That is to say, the marginal resources that we apply to health care result in tangible benefits that justify the expenditure of those resources. Enthoven and Kronick predicted that if adopted on a national scale, managed competition would lead to "a restructured market system in which the efficient prosper and the inefficient must improve or fail" (Enthoven and Kronick 1991). Such a state of equilibrium in the market for health care would, they argue, place reasonable limits on the cost of our health care system.

Historically our health care system has embodied a number of financial incentives to provide more care than is necessary, resulting in substantial inefficiency in our system of care. These incentives include the tax treatment of health insurance premiums and the system of paying physicians a separate fee for each service provided regardless of the added benefits of that service. These incentives lead to patients expecting and physicians providing a great deal of expensive care with relatively little marginal benefit. Given the opportunity to operate without these and other perverse incentives previously embodied in tax laws and laws regulating medical practice, the market will tend to weed out inefficient providers of care. Whether they provide care that is of high cost or low quality, or simply provide poor service to their patients, health care organizations that are not able to operate efficiently will not survive in a system based on managed competition. By creating a system of competing organizations—large purchasers on the demand side and managed care organizations on the supply side—the market would select for those organizations and organizational forms that operate efficiently, and in so doing will ensure the provision of cost-effective, high-quality care. This belief in market efficiency forms the theoretical core of managed competition proposals. The theory behind managed competition predicts that if a properly structured market were created, "the health care system would be transformed, gradually and voluntarily, from today's system with built-in cost-increasing incentives to a system with built-in incentives for consumer satisfaction and cost control" (Enthoven 1980, p. xxii).

Putting Managed Competition into Action: The Clinton Health Reform Proposal

During the presidential election campaign in 1992, Bill Clinton promised that if elected, he would move rapidly to reform the United States system of health care. Shortly after assuming office, he took steps to put this plan in action. In doing so he made a policy decision that a number of authors suggest was fundamentally flawed (Johnson and Broder 1996; Skocpol 1997). Rather than relying on the process of congressional hearings to arrive at a final plan for reform, he chose to create a task force of experts within the executive branch, under the supervision of First Lady Hillary Clinton. He charged this task force with developing a comprehensive, detailed plan for national health care reform.

The plan developed by the task force and presented to Congress had at its core Enthoven's theory of managed competition. The Clinton plan differed from the plan proposed by Enthoven in a number of important ways.

1. The Clinton plan proposed that each state establish a single, statewide, publicly financed HIPC, and that all residents of the state obtain their health coverage through the HIPC. Enthoven sees HIPCs as much smaller, with one for each region within a state.

2. The Clinton plan allowed employers with at least 5000 employees to act as their own HIPC. The Enthoven plan would allow employers with 1000 employees this option.

3. The Clinton plan relied on a national health board to establish the benefits that must be included in the basic benefit plan. The Enthoven plan left this decision up to the HIPCs and the market.

4. The Clinton plan gave the national health board the authority to regulate the rates that managed care plans could charge HIPCs for the basic benefit package. The Enthoven plan left the setting of rates up to the market and to competition among managed care providers.

A number of other plans were proposed in Congress as alternatives to the Clinton plan. Many of these alternatives also relied on the theory of managed competition, but with less government authority to regulate care. It appeared that after more than 10 years of discussion and debate, the time had finally come to adopt managed competition as our national policy of care. Kingdon's "window of opportunity" for major national health care reform seemed to be open.

History, however, would prove otherwise. While President Clinton was taking more than a year to formulate the specifics of his plan, the political tide in the United States shifted dramatically. The Republican Party in Congress, under the leadership of Representative Newt Gingrich, sensed that President Clinton and the Democrats had exposed their Achilles' heel. The plan offered by the Clinton administration sounded a lot like another "big government" solution to a social problem, typical of many of the failed solutions of the 1960s War on Poverty. Through a series of parliamentary procedures, the Republicans were able to stall consideration of health care reform. During this time the health insurance industry, feeling threatened by proposals to transfer the purchasing of health insurance from them to HIPCs, ran an amazingly effective series of TV ads attacking the Clinton proposal. These "Harry and Louise" ads portrayed a typical white, middle-class couple who were afraid that they were going to lose their health insurance and have to accept coverage provided by an immense government bureaucracy. Even though the claims of these ads were of tenuous accuracy, they hit home with American consumers. The combination of the Republican stalling tactics and the fear of government bureaucracy in health care engendered by Harry and Louise shifted the political landscape almost overnight. The political circumstances were no longer amenable to change. The three conditions identified by Kingdon no longer existed. The window of opportunity for national health care reform slammed shut. The Clinton plan was defeated, and the new Republican congressional leaders made it abundantly clear there was little if any chance for health care reform in the foreseeable future.

The Shift to For-Profit, Managed Care: The Market Does What the Government Would Not

Even though Congress failed to enact national health care reform, nonetheless a fundamental shift took place in the 1990s in our health care system. This shift had many, but not all, of the characteristics of managed competition as proposed by Enthoven. The rapidly rising cost of care, coupled with the growing awareness of the concept of managed care engendered by the debate over the Clinton plan, led many employers to turn to managed care to control the cost of providing care to their employees. In addition, employers have banded together in some parts of the country to establish purchasing cooperatives for health care, as envisioned by the original theory of managed competition. A number of these HIPCs have been quite successful in holding down the price of health coverage by getting the various available health plans to compete among themselves to offer the lowest price. An example of such a private, employer-sponsored HIPC is the Pacific Business Group on Health (PBGH), established by many of the biggest employers in California. All these employers chose to offer their employees only those health insurance plans approved by PBGH, at capitation rates negotiated by PBGH. Representing hundreds of thousands of potential health plan enrollees, PBGH has been very effective in negotiating low rates for health plan coverage. Few managed care providers were willing to forgo the opportunity of enrolling PBGH members. To do so would mean the potential loss of thousands of health plan members. From the 10–15% yearly increases in health plan rates seen in the early 1990s, PBGH was able in many cases to negotiate actual reductions in rates from many managed care providers. For several years in a row the cost of providing care to employees leveled out for the employers composing PBGH. Managed competition seemed to work, at least in some contexts.

Other groups had similar success in holding down the cost of care by adopting the competitive model of managed competition. Notable among these were large, governmentally supported organizations that provided health coverage for public sector employees such as the California Public

Employees Retirement System (CalPERS) and the Federal Employees Health Benefits Plan (FEHBP). In the mid-1990s they too experienced a dramatic leveling in the cost of providing coverage to their members.

In the face of the success of these large purchasing cooperatives, organized on the model of HIPCs, the economics of the entire health care system in the United States changed during the 1990s. Employers and managed care plans not involved in formally structured HIPCS were able to reduce the rate at which the cost of care was increasing. Even Medicare and Medicaid began to look to managed care and managed competition as a potential solution to the rising costs of these programs.

The 1990s saw the movement to managed care among the general public, the rise of powerful HIPCs such as PBGH, CalPERS, and FEHBP, the opening up of Medicare to managed care, and the growing conversion to managed Medicaid. Over the period of only a few years our national health care system changed to one based largely on managed care. An overwhelming majority of Americans covered by health insurance today are covered under one form of managed care or another. By 1998 there were 1037 PPOs and 647 HMOs in the country (data from the American Association of Health Plans). Even without national legislation actually mandating a shift to managed care and managed competition, the private marketplace for health insurance brought this model about.

Concept 7.3

Despite the failure of the United States Congress to enact national health care reform during the 1990s, market forces have acted to fundamentally restructure our system of health insurance. Most people in the United States with health insurance are now covered by some form of managed care plan.

Concerns About the Effects of Managed Care and Managed Competition

The rapid movement to managed care has raised three major areas of concern that have not yet been fully understood or addressed.

1. Will managed care and managed competition actually decrease health care costs in the long term?
2. What will be the effect of managed care and managed competition on the quality of care?
3. What will be the effect of adding the profit motive to health care?

We examine each of these concerns in the remainder of this chapter.

Will Managed Care and Managed Competition Actually Decrease Health Care Costs in the Long Term?

A number of scholars in fields such as economics, political science, and sociology question the ultimate ability of market forces alone to achieve the efficient provision of socially important goods such as health care. The concern is that broad social institutions will inhibit the market's ability to attain efficiency.

As described in Chapter 2, institutions provide the rules, both formal and informal, that govern action within a society. Douglas North was awarded the Nobel Prize in economics for his work showing how market efficiency is constrained by the institutional context in which the market exists. North predicts that problems may arise when the set of institutional forces that constitute economic markets overlaps with institutions reflecting broader social and political phenomena. This interaction of social and economic institutions may impair efficient economic activity.

> *If political and economic markets were efficient . . . then the choices made would always be efficient. . . . [However], institutions . . . are always a mixed bag of those that increase and those that decrease productivity. (North 1986, p. 8)*

In numerous instances, inefficient institutions have come to predominate in American business even in the face of market forces. Take for example the standard computer keyboard, which begins with the letters QWERTY. This has been the standard keyboard configuration of typewriters and computers for decades, yet it is a relatively inefficient way to arrange the keys (David 1985). This inefficient institution has come to exist despite the effects of market forces.

Many types of institutional forces inhibit the ability of markets to achieve efficiency. These countervailing forces frequently have to do with social belief systems and generally accepted rules of behavior that are not necessarily rationally or scientifically derived. These institutional constraints on market efficiency can be formalized, as in laws and regulations, or can exert their influence informally, as with social norms and professional ethics. They derive from a number of sources, both within the market itself and from the social context in which the market exists.

Chapter 2 describes the technological imperative and other institutions affecting health care in the United States. The effects of these institutions distinguish our system of health care from that in Canada and other developed countries. They also make it very difficult to constrain the growth of medical technology and the inevitable increase in costs inherent in such growth.

Institutions such as these all too often are not economically efficient, at least in the way economists approach the concept. The market's ability to improve efficiency, the basis of the economic theory behind managed competition, is constrained by the institutions that surround it.

Even under a fully capitated, competitive system it is unlikely that managed care plans will be able to overcome many of the inefficient institutions that add so much to the cost of care. In order to attain a meaningful, long-term stabilization in the cost of care they must reduce the number of services they provide, especially expensive inpatient and other types of specialized care. To do this they must attempt to alter the behavior of the physicians practicing within their system and the expectations of patients. Public perceptions of what constitutes appropriate care exist in response to the institutions that predominate in the broader social context.

There is little doubt that care provided under capitation systems costs less than comparable care under fee-for-service systems. However, the effects of capitation on the cost of care may be limited. Managed care systems are able to eliminate certain types of inefficiencies within a given institutional context, but they may be powerless to change the surrounding context itself. Constraining the rapid escalation of technology, minimizing local variations in patterns of care, and coping with defensive medicine are no less a problem for successful managed care plans than they are for their fee-for-service competitors. Managed care and managed competition, while achieving improvements through altered financial incentives, may not be able to overcome the broad inertia of inefficient institutions. In the words of Victor Fuchs (1993, p. 1679),

> The market is a powerful and flexible instrument for allocating most goods and services, but it cannot create an equitable, universal system of insurance, cannot harness technologic change in medicine, and cannot cope with the potentially unlimited demand for health care by the elderly.

Figure 7.2 represents the long-term relationship between the cost of health care in the traditional fee-for-service system and in managed care organizations such as HMOs. Although there is a clear cost advantage for the managed care organization, this advantage has remained relatively constant over time. Both fee-for-service and managed care delivery systems must contend with broad social forces that seem inexorably to drive up the cost of care.

The theory of managed competition predicts that by shifting from fee-for-service to a system of competing managed care organizations, we can arrest the increasing cost of care. This goal will be obtained by weeding out the inefficiencies inherent in fee-for-service.

Looking at the cost of care in the United States measured as a percentage of GDP spent on health care, it appears that this prediction was accu-

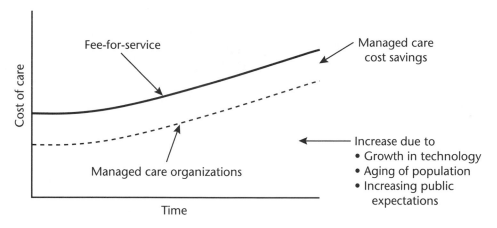

Figure 7.2 Managed Care and the Rising Cost of Care

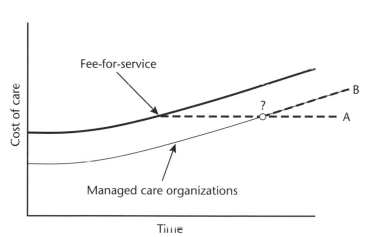

Figure 7.3 Can Managed Care Stop the Rising Cost of

rate. Between 1993 and 1998, the period when managed care became the norm in the United States, health care expenditures remained relatively constant, averaging 13.6% of GDP.

What, though, will happen when the transition to managed care is complete? Will the cost of care remain level, or will the rise in the cost of care resume? Figure 7.3 illustrates this question.

The theory of managed competition predicts that the cost of care will remain level, illustrated by the line labeled A in Figure 7.3. If, however, managed care organizations face the same institutional forces driving up the cost of care that affect the fee-for-service system, the cost savings of a national shift to managed care will be a one-time phenomenon. Once the cost of care bumps up against the managed care curve in Figure 7.3, it will resume its yearly increase at the same rate as before. This outcome is illustrated by the line labeled B.

From data that are beginning to become available it appears that outcome B more accurately represents the future of health care in America, at
least for the foreseeable future. The federal government's Health Care
Financing Administration (HCFA) predicts that after a six-year hiatus, the
cost of care will again begin to increase at a rate that is similar to the rate of
increase before 1993. HCFA predicts that the cost of health care will
increase to 15.4% in 2004 and 16.2% in 2008.

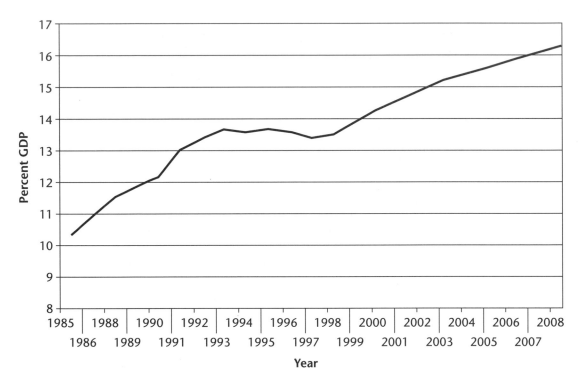

Figure 7.4 U.S. Health Care Expenditures as Percentage of GDP,
1985 –1998 (Actual) and 1999–2008 (Projected)
Source: HCFA

Figure 7.4 shows the pattern that health care costs will have taken
between 1985 and 2008 if HCFA predictions prove to be accurate. It should
be apparent that the data represented there look precisely like line B in Figure 7.3. Our health care system appears to have shifted from the fee-for-
service curve to the managed care curve without changing the actual slope
of either curve. If current predictions prove to be accurate, the theory
behind the shift to managed care will have failed the test of time.

Concept 7.4

The move to managed care that took place in this country in the 1980s and 1990s appears to have realized a one-time savings in the amount we spend on health care, but appears to have failed to arrest the long-term growth in the overall cost of health care.

What Will Be the Effect of Managed Care and Managed Competition on the Quality of Care?

In Chapter 4 we saw that there is a large difference in cost of HMO versus fee-for-service care but little difference in the health of patients treated under the two systems. One would therefore expect little adverse effect on overall health outcomes as a result of the shift to managed care experienced during the 1990s.

Figure 2.2 illustrated that much of the care we receive in this country may offer little added benefit relative to the added cost of that care. The way that managed care saves money (at least in theory) is by providing less care that has a poor marginal benefit/marginal cost ratio. Many of the control mechanisms built into managed care delivery systems approach the provision of care from this perspective.

Managed care organizations have developed a variety of mechanisms to control the cost of care to members and thus stay within their yearly budget. Some of the more common mechanisms are described below.

Gatekeepers In many managed care organizations, patients must first see their primary care physician before they can consult a specialist, get a test, or be admitted to the hospital. Patients can choose their own primary care physician, but only from among those belonging to the medical group selected by the member. In addition, once patients are referred to a specialist by the primary care physician, they are not free to select their own specialist. They usually must go to the one chosen by the primary care physician.

There are two ways the gatekeeper approach can be used.

1. The primary care physician has no direct financial stake in whether a patient is referred to a specialist or for a test. The physician's only financial interest is in maintaining the economic health of the medical group.

2. The primary care physician gets a fixed amount of money to provide all outpatient care and tests for each patient in the practice. Every time the physician refers a patient to a specialist or gets a test, the money to pay for it comes from this pool of money. Whatever is left in the pool at the end of the month is the physician's salary for that month. (Although

common during the early days of managed care, linking the gatekeeper function directly to the physician's income creates an obvious ethical conflict that has made this type of arrangement much less common.)

Utilization Review Many managed care companies maintain a staff of physicians and nurses who review the care provided by physicians. To hospitalize a patient or get an expensive test such as an MRI, the physician must obtain permission from the utilization review department. Failure to obtain this prior authorization for nonemergency treatments and procedures may lead to the managed care company refusing to pay for the service. Once a patient has been hospitalized, the utilization review staff reviews the patient's progress and makes sure the doctor doesn't keep the patient in the hospital too long.

Physician Practice Profiles Many managed care companies gather statistics on how often each physician uses expensive resources such as MRIs, expensive drugs, hospitals, and operations. The company may then penalize physicians whose profile exceeds what the reviewers think is appropriate. In a number of cases managed care companies have terminated the contracts of physicians who continually exceed expectations in the services they provide.

Financial Incentives Managed care companies have developed a variety of financial incentives intended to encourage physicians to reduce the amount of care they provide. Several examples are listed below.

Holdbacks: Managed care companies that pay physicians on a fee-for-service basis (for example, IPA HMOs) often hold back a portion of the payment due to the physician, typically 10–15%. This money is held in a reserve account for each physician. If the medical group the physician belongs to (often an IPA with hundreds of members) provides more care, in aggregate, than the managed care company has budgeted, the money to cover the cost overruns comes out of the pool of physicians' heldback pay. Physicians will receive only their portion of the holdback pool that is left over at the end of the year.

Direct bonus: Under many managed care contracts, each physician may receive a cash bonus at the end of the year, typically several thousand dollars. The amount of the bonus is determined by how well that physician has kept down costs during the year. Each physician's bonus is tied directly to the cost of the care that physician has ordered during the year.

Indirect bonus: In many medical groups that treat patients on a capitation basis, any surplus funds left over at the end of the year are placed in a bonus pool. Each physician in the group will get a share of the pool in the form of a yearly bonus. Contrary to the direct bonus, in which the amount is tied directly to the individual physician's treatment decisions, the indirect bonus is tied to the ability of the medical group as a whole to hold down costs.

A consensus appears to have developed that the indirect bonus provides a more ethical type of financial incentive to physicians. It gives each physician a stake in the financial health of the overall medical group without tying bonuses directly to the physicians' specific treatment decisions during the year.

Education and Feedback A number of medical groups that have assumed capitated risk for their patients have initiated structured programs of education and feedback to remind physicians which types of care are most appropriate and which types may be inappropriate.

In the face of utilization control mechanisms such as these, public concern has grown about maintaining the quality of care provided under managed care. Both physicians and patients often approach quality in health care as reflecting both the process of care and the outcomes from care. Care that does not meet expectations regarding process can easily be perceived as low-quality care, even if health outcomes are maintained. Take for example the treatment of ankle injuries. There is ample scientific evidence that certain, types of ankle injuries have an extremely low likelihood of involving injury to the bone. Taking X rays of these patients will add substantial cost with little or no change in the eventual healing of the injury. Nonetheless many patients who seek treatment for an injured ankle believe that unless the doctor gets an X ray, the quality of care has been substandard.

This focus on process over outcomes in defining quality has become increasingly common as more and more patients experience managed care. News reports have included numerous instances of patients being denied care that seems appropriate. Whether it is CAT scans for headaches, MRIs for knee injuries, hospitalization, referral to a specialist, use of the latest antibiotic, or access to surgery, many patients come away from their interaction with managed care systems believing that they have been denied appropriate care simply to save money. In the minds of many people, managed care means low-quality care.

The rising public outcry over the limitations that are inherent in managed care has led to increasing scrutiny of managed care organizations. Many employers and other large purchasers of care now insist that managed care providers provide comprehensive data regarding the quality of the care they provide. The most prevalent data tool used to assess quality is the Health Employers Data Information Set (HEDIS), a detailed reporting of adherence to certain process standards in care. (As with other monitoring tools, HEDIS does little to assess actual health outcomes.)

The federal government and many state governments have begun to take steps to monitor and control the quality of care provided by managed care organizations. A growing list of actual or proposed legislation has begun to define what have come to be called "patients' rights" regarding health care. Proposals talk about a "right to see a specialist," a "right to have emergency room care paid for," and a "right to appeal a denial of care."

(It is especially ironic that both government and the public are beginning to refer to "patients' rights" to care. As discussed in Chapter 1, the United States historically has failed to acknowledge a right to health care, a policy position that is unique among developed countries. As a society we appear to be defining a right to expensive, often high-tech care for those with health insurance, while denying a right even to basic care for those without health insurance. See Chapter 10 for further discussion of this issue.)

The conflict between patients' expectations of care and the need of managed care organizations to constrain care in order to control costs often places the physician directly in the middle. Physicians often find themselves in the role of wanting to provide a certain service or type of care but having the managed care company refusing to authorize or pay for care. Medical meetings and newsletters frequently bemoan the added burden that has been placed on physicians by managed care. Doctors describe spending hours on the phone with managed care reviewers (most of them with no medical training) debating the necessity of a certain type of care. Many doctors complain that clinical decision making has been taken out of their hands and placed in the hands of bureaucrats.

Many of these complaints and concerns about the effect of managed care on quality are in response to actions that have substantial scientific support. From the perspective of managed care companies, it makes little sense to pay for a service that will have little or no added benefit when measured in terms of health outcomes. When a doctor asks for approval to undertake a procedure that has been shown to have little benefit in carefully controlled, scientific studies, it is both understandable and defensible to deny coverage for that care. This is precisely how HMOs and other managed care organizations save money. Nonetheless, the public response to denials of this type is often one of criticism and complaint over low-quality care. It appears that managed care as a means of controlling health care costs (the basic reason our system of care has turned to it so completely) has a fundamental inconsistency. Unless the institutions and belief systems inherent in our society change regarding what constitutes high-quality care, any success that managed care achieves in holding down the cost of care is at risk of being seen as a decrease in the quality of care.

There is one important caveat to this conclusion. As discussed in the following section, the move to for-profit organizations as the basic organi-

> ### Concept 7.5
>
> Many of the reductions in care initiated by managed care companies in an effort to control costs have come to be perceived by the public as unwarranted reductions in quality.

zational model of our system has superimposed concerns about the profit motive on top of concerns about the quality of care.

What Will Be the Effect of Adding the Profit Motive to Health Care?

Throughout most of the twentieth century there was little room in our health care delivery system for for-profit organizations. Although a number of for-profit insurance companies offered health insurance as one of their products, the predominant model for health insurance was the Blue Cross/Blue Shield system, organized on a nonprofit basis. Physicians often practiced as professional corporations, but few worked for or managed practice organizations that operated on a for-profit basis.

Hospitals traditionally have run on a nonprofit basis in the United States. After the enactment of Medicare and Medicaid, many doctors and businessmen saw the potential of operating hospitals as moneymaking businesses. Beginning in the 1970s, investor-owned, for-profit corporations began to purchase hospitals and other types of institutional care facilities. Using capital obtained through the sale of stock, corporations took over formerly nonprofit hospitals and began to run them on a for-profit basis. Many people were concerned that this shift to a for-profit orientation in the provision of health care created potential problems, including

Ethical problems for physicians revolving around conflict of interest (Would physicians have to choose between making money for the corporation and doing what is best for the patient?)

The effects on the autonomy of doctors and other professionals (Would business managers end up telling doctors what they could and couldn't do?)

The goals and policies that for-profit hospitals would adopt (Would for-profit hospitals ignore local community needs and exploit employees?)

The effects on medical research and education (Would for-profit hospitals benefit from publicly financed research and educational programs without contributing to them?)

A number of eyebrows were raised in the medical community over these and other concerns. In 1986 the Institute of Medicine, a branch of the federal National Academy of Sciences, looked into the effect of for-profit care in hospitals and issued a report (Gray 1986). The report found that when compared to traditional nonprofit hospitals, for-profit hospitals are slightly less efficient in producing a given service or procedure, charge somewhat more for comparable services, and provide less uncompensated care to low-income patients. They also have been able to raise capital for expansion more easily than nonprofit hospitals. (For-profit hospitals raise capital through issuing stock; nonprofit hospitals raise capital by borrowing it.)

The report found no data available to compare the actual quality of the care at for-profit and nonprofit hospitals. It did raise the question of whether for-profit hospitals "skim" the patient population, that is treat only those patients with good insurance who can pay for their care, thus leaving the unprofitable patients for the nonprofit hospitals. If this were indeed the case, it would mean that nonprofit hospitals are having to face an increased financial burden because of the selective policies of the for-profit hospitals.

Some arguments have also been offered in favor of for-profit hospitals:

For-profit hospital systems have the potential to provide care more efficiently if managed well; financial incentives could be structured to support efficient care.

Competition among for-profit and nonprofit hospitals will, in theory, weed out inefficient systems of care, thus reducing overall costs.

The initial movement of for-profit corporations into hospital ownership did not have a substantial effect on the overall health care system. The actual financing of care, whether by insurance companies or managed care organizations, remained largely a nonprofit activity throughout much of the 1980s. However, in the early 1990s for-profit health care companies received huge infusions of cash from the booming American stock market. For-profit corporations began increasingly to appear in many segments of the health care system, including the following four.

Hospitals The somewhat lackluster growth of earlier, for-profit hospital chains was quickly overshadowed by the exponential growth of newer organizations. Chief among these was Columbia-HCA, a huge hospital conglomerate that seemed to spring up overnight. With cash provided by the sale of stock, Columbia-HCA bought up formerly nonprofit hospitals in many parts of the country, and for a while seemed headed toward becoming the predominant owner of hospitals in the country.

Physician Practice Management Organizations (PPMs) A number of physicians in small, office-based practice felt seriously threatened by the rapid shift to managed care, unable to compete for patients and cope with the growing limitations on care. A number of business entrepreneurs (many of them physicians) recognized an opportunity, and offered to come to the aid of the beleaguered doctors. With money raised through the sale of stock, these businessmen offered to buy out the practice of both individual doctors and small groups of doctors, and to hire the doctor back as an employee. For many doctors the offer was irresistible. They would receive a substantial sum of cash, they could continue to treat their own patients, and they wouldn't have to cope with the hassle of managed care. Many doctors readily turned the operation of their practice over to for-profit PPMs. Problems quickly developed, and many of the doctors did not take well to their new role as employee. They lost substantial operational control over their office, over the personnel who worked under them, and over which patients they would see. Increases in income offered by the PPMs as incentive to sell often failed to materialize. Tension sometimes bordering on open conflict developed between physicians and their PPM owners.

Medical Specialty Companies The growing role of high-tech treatment in many areas of medicine presented an opportunity for physicians in certain areas of practice to become businessmen as well as clinicians. With money obtained through the sale of stock it was quite easy to develop specialized, for-profit facilities such as kidney dialysis centers, cancer treatment centers, or outpatient surgery centers. These for-profit centers are becoming increasingly prevalent in many areas of medical practice.

Managed Care Organizations With the removal of the requirement in the 1980s that HMOs be operated on a nonprofit basis, the for-profit HMO became an increasingly important part of our health system. Especially under the group-model HMO described in Chapter 4, it was often quite straightforward for small corporations to raise cash from the stock market, establish a network of hospitals and physician groups, and offer coverage through this network to employers. As regional, for-profit HMOs developed in many areas of the country, other, larger HMOs would often move in and buy them up, creating in the process very large networks of providers. For these new HMOs and other types of managed care organizations, the name of the game was market share. It was crucial to their success that they rapidly establish a substantial presence in the market, measured by the number of patients enrolled in their plans. To achieve this goal many companies priced their coverage artificially low, making them especially attractive to employers and employees. By 1998 nearly two-thirds of all patients enrolled in HMOs nationwide were in for-profit HMOs.

As the market became increasingly competitive, though, many companies found it difficult to raise prices once their presence in the market had been established. Facing the potential of large financial losses, many of these companies began to put increasing pressure on the physicians and hospitals with which they contracted to hold down the cost of care. Many of the practices of managed care companies that led to the patients' rights movement and to physician consternation were initiated by for-profit companies.

The health insurance industry has coined a somewhat odd phrase: the "medical loss ratio" (MLR). The MLR is simply the percentage of every dollar taken in as insurance premiums that goes to pay the direct cost of providing care. An MLR of 90% would mean that 90% of every premium dollar goes to pay for medical care. The remaining 10% would go to cover activities not involved directly in patient care such as marketing, administrative overhead, and shareholder dividend. The phrase is odd because it implies that health insurance companies, in business to provide health insurance, consider any funds actually spent providing care to patients to be a loss.

Historically the MLR of nonprofit HMOs such as Kaiser-Permanente has been in the range of 95%. If one calculates the MLR for the Medicare and Medicaid programs, they typically are between 95% and 98%. Nearly all of the money in these traditional programs goes to pay for care.

In the new world of for-profit managed care, MLRs typically range from 70% to 85%. Any for-profit company that maintains an MLR above 80% is at a potentially serious competitive disadvantage. Their disadvantage, though, is not in competing for patients but rather in competing for stock market investment. In the face of rising cost pressures in medicine, companies that are unable to maintain low MLRs will have difficulty giving shareholders an adequate return on their investment. Managers of these companies will be facing possible termination due to poor stock performance.

Adding the profit motive and the pressure to maintain a low MLR to the cost pressures inherent in all managed care has compounded the negative public reaction to the managed care industry. These pressures may be partially responsible for the lower quality of care that has been shown to exist in some for-profit HMOs. Using HEDIS scores as a measure of quality, a recent study demonstrated that the for-profit HMOs included in the study maintained significantly lower levels of quality than their nonprofit competitors (Himmelstein et al. 1999).

Neither the public nor legislators seem able to separate problems in quality that stem from the profit motive and perceived problems that stem from efforts to control unnecessary care. The negative reaction to the managed care industry has been remarkably uniform and widespread, and seems to have lumped these two issues together. Only time will tell whether the combination of for-profit corporations and managed care will be able to survive in its current form.

One thing that is clear is that in this increasingly critical and competitive climate, investors have begun to lose interest in for-profit health care companies, sometimes with disastrous results for the companies. After years of high-flying success, Columbia-HCA has had to face a combination of growing losses and federal probes of possible fraud. Physician practice management organizations have had severe difficulties, with many of them going out of business. A number of large, for-profit HMOs have faced huge financial losses. After maintaining average annual returns of 38% between 1988 and 1995, for-profit HMOs averaged an 11% yearly loss between 1995 and 1997. Other health service companies faced similar problems, going from annual returns averaging 23% between 1988 and 1995 to annual losses averaging 19%. The continued ability of for-profit health care companies to raise money in the stock market faces serious questions.

Concept 7.6

The widespread move to for-profit health care, and the need to maintain shareholder profits inherent in that move, have created additional pressures on the health care system to hold down costs. The expansion of for-profit care has compounded the public's negative reaction to managed care, creating the "managed care backlash."

REFERENCES

American Association of Health Plans. Enrollment, Growth, Accreditation. October 1999, available at www.aahp.org/.

Arrow K. Uncertainty and the Welfare Economics of Medical Care. *American Economic Review* 1963; 53:941–69.

David PA. Clio and the Economics of QWERTY. *AEA Papers and Proceedings* 1985; 75:332.

Enthoven A. *Health Plan: The Only Practical Solution to the Soaring Cost of Medical Care.* Reading, Mass.: Addison-Wesley, 1980.

Enthoven AE, Kronick R. A Consumer-Choice Health Plan for the 1990s. *New England Journal of Medicine* 1989; 320:29–37, 94–101.

Enthoven AE, Kronick R. Universal Health Insurance Through Incentives Reform. *JAMA* 1991; 265:2532–36.

Fuchs VR. Dear President Clinton. *JAMA* 1993; 269:1678–79.

Gray B. *For-Profit Enterprise in Health Care*. Washington, D.C. : National Academy Press, 1986.

Himmelstein DU, Woolhandler S, Hellander I, Wolfe SM. Quality of Care in Investor-Owned vs Not-for-Profit HMOs. *JAMA* 1999; 282:159–63.

Johnson H, Broder DS. *The System*. Boston: Little, Brown, 1996.

Kaiser Family Foundation. For-Profit Health Care Companies: Trends and Issues. May 8, 2000, available at http://www.kff.org/content/archive/1359/facts.html

Kingdon JW. *Agendas, Alternatives, and Public Policies*. Boston: Little, Brown, 1984.

North DC. *Institutions, Institutional Change and Economic Performance*. New York: Cambridge University Press, 1986.

Skocpol T. *Boomerang—Health Care Reform and the Turn Against Government*. New York: W.W. Norton, 1997.

CHAPTER 8

Recent Changes to the Medicare Program

Key Concepts

- In an attempt to reduce program costs, Medicare created the option for beneficiaries to enroll in certain approved HMOs. Because most of these Medicare HMOs offered benefits not provided by traditional Medicare, they proved to be very successful in enrolling large numbers of beneficiaries.

- If a managed care health plan is able to enroll members who, on average, are healthier than the general population, it has benefited from *favorable selection*. If a plan finds that it has enrolled members who, on average, are sicker than the general population, it has suffered from *adverse selection*.

- Data gathered by the HCFA have shown that most Medicare HMOs benefited from substantial favorable selection in the enrollment of beneficiaries.

- The Balanced Budget Act of 1997 added several new alternatives for Medicare beneficiaries to obtain care, referred to collectively as "Medicare + Choice." The intent was to reduce the long-term costs of Medicare by introducing a larger role for market forces.

- The Balanced Budget Act of 1997 had a number of adverse consequences that Congress had not intended. Among these were a large-scale exodus of many HMOs from the Medicare program and severe financial hardship for many hospitals.

As previous chapters have discussed, the 1980s and 1990s were periods of rapid change in American health care. As the cost of care began to skyrocket, employers and other large purchasers of health insurance turned to HMOs and other types of managed care delivery systems. The number of Americans receiving their care from managed care organizations increased by several orders of magnitude.

During this time the federal government experienced the same cost pressures as businesses. As shown in Figure 5.5, the cost of the Medicare program increased dramatically between 1977 and 1997. Administrators at the federal government's Health Care Financing Administration (HCFA) began to look to HMOs as potential solutions to the problem of rising costs. As early as 1976 Congress took steps to allow Medicare beneficiaries to enroll in HMOs as an alternative to traditional Medicare coverage. As the costs of Medicare continued to increase despite previous efforts to contain them, the federal government took several steps to reform the program. A number of these steps have been quite controversial. Not all have worked as intended. This chapter discusses the changes in Medicare that were initiated in the 1990s, the period of the managed care revolution.

The Initial Move to Medicare HMOs: Getting More for Less for Medicare Beneficiaries

Starting in the 1970s, the federal government began to pay HMOs enrolling Medicare beneficiaries based on cost reimbursement. The HMO would keep track of the cost of providing care to the beneficiary and HCFA would reimburse a portion of that cost. This policy of cost reimbursement provided little incentive for the HMO to constrain the use of services for beneficiaries and did little to reduce Medicare costs. Accordingly, in the early 1980s HCFA switched from enrolling Medicare beneficiaries in HMOs on a cost basis to enrolling them on a risk basis.

Establishing Risk-Contracting with HMOs

Medicare needed a way to take advantage of the potential cost savings that appeared to be inherent in HMOs. HCFA created a new way of paying HMOs that shifted most of the risk for cost overruns to the HMO yet provided the HMO with an incentive to control costs. HCFA estimated that, on average, an HMO should be able to take care of a Medicare beneficiary for about 95% of what it costs to take care of beneficiaries in traditional, fee-for-service Medicare. A well-run HMO might even be able to provide care for less than 95%.

In 1985 HCFA created a policy under which any HMO that enrolled a Medicare beneficiary would be paid a yearly capitation fee that was equal to 95% of the average cost of providing care to the other beneficiaries. Because the average cost of caring for a Medicare beneficiary varies substantially across different communities and different regions of the country, the 95% rate was based on the average cost of care locally. The HMO was required to provide the same range of services that were available to beneficiaries under the traditional plan. However, if the HMO could provide care for less than 95% of the average local cost, it was free to keep the difference so long as it was used either to expand services to beneficiaries or to reduce the out-of-pocket expenses required of them.

Recall from Chapter 5 that a Medicare beneficiary enrolled in both Part A and Part B still faces substantial out-of-pocket expenses. These include

- The Part A hospital deductible for each time the patient is in the hospital
- The yearly Part B $100 deductible
- 20% of all charges covered by Part B
- Extra Part B charges (up to 15% of allowable charges) of doctors who don't accept assignment

In addition there are a variety of things that traditional Medicare simply doesn't cover, including prescription drugs, dental care, eyeglasses, hearing aids, and foot care. In order to provide insurance coverage for these added expenses, most Medicare beneficiaries obtain supplemental insurance coverage (medigap policies), often costing the beneficiary more than $1000 per year.

HMOs initially reacted favorably to the risk-contracting option. By 1987, 161 HMOs had signed risk contracts with HCFA allowing them to enroll Medicare beneficiaries. Following this initial enthusiasm were several years of confusion and uncertainty, with the number of contracting HMOs falling to 93 in 1991.

The early 1990s saw the rapid expansion of HMOs in many areas of the country. As the number of HMOs increased, the number of HMOs willing to enter risk contracts also increased. States like California, Florida, Pennsylvania, New York, and Texas saw both an increase in HMOs operating in the market and HMOs contracting with HCFA. By 1997, 307 HMOs nationwide had signed Medicare risk contracts.

Most of the HMOs enrolling Medicare patients found that the cost of providing care for their Medicare enrollees was below the 95% capitation rate. Accordingly they began to expand the types of services they provided to these enrollees. By 1995 half of all plans offered Medicare beneficiaries supplemental coverage for prescription drugs, 86% provided routine eye exams, 65% provided hearing exams, and 33% provided foot care. Most of the time these added services were at no extra charge to the beneficiary. In fact, the cost to the beneficiary was often less than traditional Medicare, even before taking into account the cost of medigap coverage.

Table 8.1   Options for Medicare Beneficiaries Under Managed Care

Traditional Medicare	Medicare HMO
Disadvantages	**Advantages**
Part A deductible	No deductible
Part B deductible	No deductible
Part B copayment	$5-per-visit copayment
No coverage for prescription drugs	Coverage for prescription drugs
No coverage for eyeglasses	Coverage for eyeglasses
Advantages	**Disadvantages**
Free choice of any physician or hospital	Choice of physician only with the health plan
No referral necessary for specialty care	Specialty care only by referral

Source: HCFA

Table 8.1 illustrates the choice offered to Medicare beneficiaries. Recall that traditional Medicare beneficiaries had to purchase their own medigap policies to cover many of the items listed in the left-hand column. Those who enrolled in a Medicare HMO that offered the supplemental coverage listed in the right-hand column did not need their medigap coverage, a substantial savings for most beneficiaries. Thus for less money than traditional Medicare, beneficiaries in HMOs were provided with substantially increased benefits. They had the option of getting more yet paying less. For many this was an option that proved hard to pass up.

By 1997 the number of Medicare beneficiaries enrolling in HMOs had increased to more than 5 million, representing nearly 15% of all beneficiaries. The number of beneficiaries enrolling in HMOs was increasing by a third or more every year. In states like California, Arizona, and Oregon, where HMOs had gained a wide share of the overall health care market, more than a third of Medicare beneficiaries had enrolled in HMOs.

Concept 8.1

In an attempt to reduce program costs, Medicare created the option for beneficiaries to enroll in certain approved HMOs. Because most of these Medicare HMOs offered benefits not provided by traditional Medicare, they proved to be very successful in enrolling large numbers of beneficiaries.

Enrolling in an HMO did have certain drawbacks for Medicare beneficiaries, mostly involving the choice of physician or hospital. Under traditional Medicare each beneficiary is able to obtain care from any physician who has registered with Medicare. Since nearly all practicing physicians in the country are registered, traditional Medicare essentially gives beneficiaries free choice of physician anywhere in the country. Similarly, beneficiaries are able to obtain hospital care at any hospital that is certified by Medicare. Thus if a beneficiary in California chooses to fly to the Mayo Clinic in Minnesota for consultation with a physician and to undergo surgery, traditional Medicare will provide the same coverage as if the beneficiary had obtained the care in her home town. Finally, under traditional Medicare, beneficiaries are free to consult a specialist without a referral. Under many HMOs, a beneficiary must first obtain a referral from her primary care physician before consulting a specialist. Once the referral has been obtained, the beneficiary is limited to those specialists who are on the HMO's list of eligible providers. Thus, even though enrolling in an HMO held a substantial cost advantage for beneficiaries, it also meant giving up a certain amount of choice in the selection of a physician or hospital. However, for those beneficiaries who had a doctor they felt comfortable with, there was very little disadvantage in enrolling in an HMO in which their doctor participated.

Problems in HMO Risk Contracting: Favorable Selection and the Average Cost of Care

Officials in HCFA closely followed the growth of Medicare HMO enrollment throughout the early and mid-1990s. As part of the risk contract, HCFA kept track of the care provided to beneficiaries enrolled in HMOs in order to determine if any cost savings realized by the HMOs were actually returned to beneficiaries in the form of added benefits. A pattern began to emerge. It appeared that HMOs were more attractive to younger, healthier Medicare beneficiaries. Beneficiaries with more serious medical problems seemed to be more likely to stay with traditional coverage.

Favorable selection refers to a situation that can exist when two or more competing health care plans are available to potential enrollees. If the plans are equally attractive to all enrollees, then the average health status of those enrolling in one plan should be approximately the same as the health status of those enrolling in the alternative plan. However, if one option is more attractive to healthier enrollees, with the second option more attractive to enrollees who on average are sicker, there will be favorable consequences for the first plan and adverse consequences for the second. Having a higher percentage of its enrollees being sicker means it will have higher costs than the competing plan.

Concept 8.2

If a managed care health plan is able to enroll members who, on average, are healthier than the general population, it has benefited from *favorable selection*.

If a plan finds that it has enrolled members who, on average, are sicker than the general population, it has suffered from *adverse selection*.

In the case of Medicare it appears that favorable selection did occur. Those selecting the HMO option were on average healthier than those remaining in traditional Medicare. This pattern raises serious questions about the entire financing structure of Medicare HMO enrollment.

Figure 8.1 illustrates the tremendous potential impact that favorable and adverse selection can have as they apply to Medicare HMOs and traditional Medicare. Using HCFA data for 1997, the graph looks at the cost of providing care to beneficiaries who are in the 25th, 50th, 75th, or 90th percentile of yearly cost. For each level it shows

- The average cost per beneficiary at this level
- 95% of the average cost of all beneficiaries
- The difference between 95% of the average cost of care and what it actually costs to provide care to a beneficiary at this level

The third figure is, in essence, the profit (or loss) that a Medicare HMO will realize if it enrolls a Medicare beneficiary whose cost of care is at the specified level.

Take for example a beneficiary at the 50th percentile of annual cost. It costs an average of $779 to provide care for this beneficiary. Ninety-five percent of the average cost of taking care of other beneficiaries is $5584, which is the amount an HMO would receive from HCFA to care for the beneficiary. The HMO would receive $4805 more than it actually costs to provide care for the beneficiary.

Now look at the beneficiary at the 90th percentile of annual cost. It takes on average $14,000 to provide care for these beneficiaries, which is $8416 *more* than the HMO actually gets paid. For approximately 80% of beneficiaries, the annual cost of care is less than the amount paid by HCFA for HMO care. For the remaining 20%, the cost of care is more than the HCFA capitation rate. If an HMO can attract more of the younger, healthier beneficiaries and fewer of the older, sicker beneficiaries, it can keep its annual cost of care for these beneficiaries substantially below the amount it receives from HCFA.

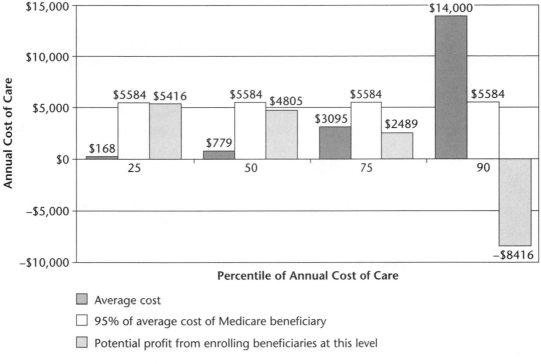

Figure 8.1 HMO Cost Compared to Capitation Rate for Medicare Beneficiaries at Four Percentiles, 1997
Source: HCFA

One additional point is worth mentioning. Recall that the 95% capitation rate was calculated based on what it costs to provide care to beneficiaries remaining with traditional Medicare. (Recall also that this figure was calculated regionally.) If, as appears to have been the case, those remaining with traditional Medicare were drawn disproportionately from the population of older and sicker beneficiaries, the cost of providing care for these remaining beneficiaries would be even higher than the overall average cost of providing care for all beneficiaries. This situation would only magnify the potential benefit of favorable selection for those HMOs who enroll younger, healthier beneficiaries.

Under the regulations established by HCFA, any surplus funds obtained through enrolling Medicare beneficiaries must be returned to the beneficiaries either in the form of lower costs or higher benefits. The HMOs who benefited from the lower costs associated with healthier beneficiaries added the benefits described above. Even with these added benefits, in many cases it still cost HMOs less to care for their beneficiaries than the capitation payment they received for providing care. These HMOs were able to increase their profits through enrolling Medicare beneficiaries. The end result was that the Medicare HMO program resulted in increased overall spending, rather than the decrease that was intended when the program was established.

Analysts within HCFA were able to build a strong case for adjusting the capitation rate paid to HMOs downward. They estimated that as a consequence of disproportionately enrolling younger, healthier beneficiaries, HMOs were facing actual costs that were approximately 5% lower than the costs initially estimated. At a time when there was a major national effort to reduce the overall federal budget deficit and control the rising cost of Medicare, the identification of actual *overpayments* to HMOs was of concern both to HCFA analysts and to members of Congress. In response to these calculations Congress was to take action that would prove to have a profound effect on the entire Medicare HMO program.

Concept 8.3

Data gathered by HCFA have shown that most Medicare HMOs benefited from substantial favorable selection in the enrollment of beneficiaries.

The Balanced Budget Act of 1997 and Its Effect on Medicare

The Balanced Budget Act of 1997 was a complex set of changes in the financing and organization of a broad range of federal policies. Medicare was only one of the topics covered in this attempt to shift the federal government from chronically spending more on programs than it received in taxes. Years of deficit spending had led to a huge federal debt. The Balanced Budget Act attempted to ensure that the federal government would balance its budget on an ongoing basis.

One of the first things the Balanced Budget Act did was to change the way that HCFA pays HMOs to enroll Medicare beneficiaries. As discussed above, for years HCFA had paid HMOs 95% of the average cost of caring for fee-for-service Medicare patients, adjusted for regional differences. The 95% payment rate was thought to be too generous, so the act cut this yearly capitation rate to about 90% of the average cost of providing care to fee-for-service Medicare beneficiaries. HCFA contended that the pattern of favorable selection that had gone on previously made the 90% figure more appropriate.

At the same time that HCFA was raising concerns about the financing structure of the Medicare HMO program, members of Congress were looking to reform Medicare in a number of additional ways. Leaders of the

Republican Party in Congress, in a position of control of both houses for the first time since Medicare was established, wanted to shift certain portions of Medicare to reflect a more market-based approach. The concept was to allow Medicare beneficiaries a wide range of choices for obtaining care in addition to traditional Medicare or a Medicare HMO. Two principal alternatives were put forward.

Medical Savings Account

The Rand Health Insurance Experiment, discussed in more detail in Chapter 11, showed that when patients are required to pay for a substantial portion of their care out of pocket, they will use less care. The concept of the medical savings account (MSA) builds on this finding. It is based on the assumption that if a Medicare beneficiary is personally responsible for the first several thousand dollars of medical care costs per year, that beneficiary will use less care, and the overall cost of care will be less. The MSA provides a modified, high-deductible Medicare plan for those beneficiaries who select it. This plan, based on the traditional fee-for-service payment method, would take effect only after the patient had met the required annual deductible. Beneficiaries can select plans with deductibles of up to $6000 per year. It can reasonably be expected that the cost of such plans would be substantially less than the cost of providing care under traditional Medicare. Under the MSA, an amount equal to the difference between the cost of the high-deductible plan and the amount Medicare would otherwise pay to enroll the beneficiary in a Medicare HMO would be placed in a savings account in the beneficiary's name. For example, if the annual premium for the high-deductible plan were $3000 and the amount available for HMO enrollment were $5800 (approximately the amount actually paid in 1998), Medicare would deposit $2800 into a savings account for use by the beneficiary. However, if the beneficiary did not use the full $2800 during the year, he would be allowed to keep the remaining balance. Initially the amount left over at the end of the year would be rolled over to the next year. Medicare would deposit an additional $2800 into the account for that next year.

Recall from Figure 8.1 that for 75% of Medicare beneficiaries the cost of providing their medical care in 1997 was $3095 or less. The majority of these beneficiaries stood a good chance of having money left over in the MSA at the end of the year for several years in a row. The amount in the MSA could easily build up. So long as the beneficiary at all times maintained an amount in the MSA equal to 60% of the yearly deductible, the beneficiary would be allowed to withdraw any additional funds and use these funds for any purpose the beneficiary chooses. Funds used in this manner would be subject to income tax.

It can be seen that an MSA might be very attractive to a Medicare beneficiary who is in excellent overall health and can reasonably expect few out-of-pocket health care expenditures. It can also be seen that for those beneficiaries with chronic medical problems and high yearly expenses, the MSA has relatively little to offer. This difference is one of the principal drawbacks to the MSA. MSAs would most likely enroll a disproportionate number of young, healthy beneficiaries, leaving the older, sicker beneficiaries in traditional Medicare. Since the amount available to pay the costs of the MSA program would be calculated as a percentage of the cost of caring for beneficiaries staying with traditional Medicare, the MSA could actually lead to higher overall costs, in a manner similar to the HMO program. Instead of cost savings in the MSA going for added health care benefits (or added profits for the HMO), in this case the savings could pay for a trip to visit the grandchildren. These aspects of the program have made the MSA difficult for many legislators to accept.

Given the uncertainty surrounding the MSA proposals, the Balanced Budget Act of 1997 created the option for up to 390,000 beneficiaries to enroll in MSAs on a trial basis. These plans will be in operation for four years, ending in 2002. HCFA will then evaluate the plans to see if they do provide a viable alternative to the traditional fee-for-service program and the Medicare HMO option.

Medicare + Choice: Expanding the Range of Managed Care Options

A number of members of Congress wanted to amend the Medicare HMO program to allow a wider range of managed care options for beneficiaries. Although the shift to managed care in the broader health care system had begun with HMOs, the 1990s had seen the proliferation of other managed care financing and delivery systems that were not strictly HMOs. (See Chapter 4 for a discussion of some of these other options.)

To many in Congress, HMOs represented a form of health care that was overly bureaucratic and that unnecessarily limited the options open to patients. The widely held belief in the ability of market forces to improve the efficiency of health care delivery led to proposals to open Medicare up to a wide variety of options that were less closely regulated by the government. The proposal was to ensure Medicare beneficiaries the range of services covered by Medicare, but to allow them the choice of market-based options beyond HMOs as an alternative. Thus the name for this new program: Medicare + Choice.

Under the Balanced Budget Act, Medicare + Choice allowed Medicare beneficiaries to select from any of the following options for their Medicare coverage:

- A Medicare HMO

- A Medicare HMO that in addition provides a point of service (POS) option

- A preferred provider organization (PPO) that allows a wide range of choice of physician and hospital and pays for care on a discounted fee-for-service basis

- A physician-hospital organization (PHO) set up by a coalition of doctors and hospitals willing to accept risk-contracting for Medicare beneficiaries

- A medical savings account (MSA)

- A traditional fee-for-service insurance plan operated by a private insurance company

- The traditional Medicare program

All of these Medicare + Choice options would be required to provide the same level of benefits as the traditional program. Like Medicare HMOs, other Medicare + Choice plans would be required to return any cost savings to beneficiaries in the form of increased benefits or lower premiums. Beneficiaries would continue to have the premium for Medicare Part B withheld from their Social Security checks. For the managed care plans under Medicare + Choice, the total out-of-pocket expenditures for beneficiaries could not exceed the average out-of-pocket expenses under the traditional plan. Beneficiaries enrolling in the private, fee-for-service option under Medicare + Choice would be subject to somewhat higher out-of-pocket expenses.

Medicare would pay a yearly premium to any of the plans eligible under Medicare + Choice calculated in the same manner as the yearly capitation payment for Medicare HMOs. It would be based on a percentage of the average cost of care for beneficiaries in traditional Medicare. The issue of favorable selection would be monitored by HCFA, and yearly premiums or capitation rates adjusted accordingly. Beneficiaries would be eligible to change plans under Medicare + Choice, but after an initial transitional period, they would have the option of changing plans only once a year.

Concept 8.4

The Balanced Budget Act of 1997 added several new alternatives for Medicare beneficiaries to obtain care, referred to collectively as Medicare + Choice. The intent was to reduce the long-term costs of Medicare by introducing a larger role for market forces.

Other Medicare Changes
in the Balanced Budget Act of 1997

The principal purpose of the Balanced Budget Act was to balance the budget. Many of the changes in the Medicare program described above were intended to widen the array of choices available to Medicare beneficiaries with little or no cost saving expected in the short run. In order to ensure that the cost of Medicare did not drag the federal government back into deficit spending, the Balanced Budget Act included a number of other changes in the way Medicare was financed. Some of the key provisions are discussed in the rest of this section.

Secure the Future of the Part A Hospital Trust Fund A number of reports in the years leading up to 1997 had predicted that the Part A Trust Fund would run out of money within a few years if nothing were done. Recall that the Trust Fund is financed through the payroll tax contributions of employers and employees. In contrast to Part B financing, which can draw on the general federal treasury if costs increase, there is no mechanism to increase funding for Part A if tax revenues are not sufficient to meet Part A expenses. The two principal categories of Part A expenses were hospital care and home health care.

The Medicare home health care benefit had initially been designed to provide a means of getting patients who were being treated in the hospital back into their home as soon as possible. Medicare would pay for a range of services provided to patients in their home, including skilled nursing care, physical therapy, occupational therapy, and assistance with activities of daily living by a home health aide. Since home health care was seen as a way of getting patients out of the hospital sooner, it seemed appropriate to place the budget for home health services under the Part A Trust Fund.

Unfortunately, experience proved to be different than predictions in home health care. Home health care was successful in its goal of improving the quality of life of homebound, elderly individuals. However, rather than providing care to recently hospitalized patients, the program ended up providing services mainly to patients who had not been in the hospital. Rather than being a substitute for hospital care, it turned out to provide services that were in addition to hospital care. Although serving millions of elderly patients, it did not appear to cut down substantially on the cost of hospital care. Allocating the cost of home health care to the Part A Trust Fund appeared to be less appropriate than initially intended.

As discussed in Chapter 9, the cost of the home health care program increased dramatically between 1989 and 1997, from $2.25 billion to nearly $17 billion. Both the number of beneficiaries receiving care and the average number of visits per beneficiary increased. These changes were a major reason why the Part A Trust Fund was threatened with insolvency. The solution included in the Balanced Budget Act was quite simple: reallocate the cost of home health services that are not associated with an episode of hospital care to Part B instead of Part A. This switch did nothing to change the cost of home health care. It simply changed the fund from which the cost of these services would come. In doing so it removed a major drain on the Trust Fund and went a long way to ensuring its long-term solvency.

The Balanced Budget Act made other changes to home health care policy that were intended to cut down on the costs of the program. It cracked down on fraud and abuse in the way agencies that provide home health care bill for their services, thus saving millions of dollars per year. It also initiated a plan to create a method of paying for home health care per episode of illness rather than per visit. This prospective payment system (PPS) for home health care is intended to have many of the same effects that the PPS system of paying for hospital care had. The Balanced Budget Act also established a PPS method of paying for care in skilled nursing facilities, although using PPS to pay for care in a skilled nursing facility has proven to be more complex than paying for home health care.

Decrease Payments to Hospitals The need to maintain the solvency of the Part A Trust Fund led Congress to reduce the amount Medicare will pay for hospital care. Recall that most hospital care is paid through the prospective payment system (PPS). Historically, as the cost of providing hospital care has risen, HCFA has increased the PPS payment for that care. Based on a political decision to reduce payments to providers as a principal means of stabilizing Medicare's financing, the Balanced Budget Act mandated that HCFA reduce payments to hospitals in a variety of ways.

The first was to keep payments under the PPS system the same in 1998 as they were in 1997, even though the actual costs faced by hospitals had gone up. For the years 1999–2002, PPS payments would rise, but at a rate that was less than the actual increase in the cost of care.

A second step was to further reduce payments to hospitals that treat large numbers of poor patients. HCFA keeps track of the percentage of poor patients treated in every hospital. Those hospitals that treat a disproportionate number of poor patients receive extra payment over and above the usual PPS payment, on the assumption that caring for poor patients can be more expensive than caring for comparable patients who are not poor. These "disproportionate-share" hospitals were thus hit twice by the Balanced Budget Act: their payments were reduced under the standard PPS reductions and a second time under the specific disproportionate share reductions.

Develop a Method to "Risk Adjust" Capitation Premiums to Medicare Managed Care Plans Analysts within HCFA, the academic community, and the business community are in substantial agreement on the need to make the capitation payments to Medicare managed care plans more in line with the need for services for the covered beneficiaries. As discussed above, the cost of providing care for a beneficiary can vary substantially. It may be possible to predict how much it will cost to provide care for an individual beneficiary or for a group of beneficiaries based on the health status of those beneficiaries. For example, a 70-year-old beneficiary with diabetes and heart disease will incur substantially more costs than a 70-year-old beneficiary with no chronic medical problems. Given adequate information about the health status of beneficiaries, it may be possible to adjust the capitation payment made to a managed care plan based on the previous health status of the beneficiary. Plans enrolling beneficiaries with better health status would receive lower capitation payments, and plans enrolling beneficiaries with worse health status would receive higher capitation payments. Altering the capitation payment in this way based on the health status of the beneficiary is referred to as "risk adjusting." Congress mandated in the Balanced Budget Act that HCFA develop a method of risk-adjusting capitation premiums for Medicare managed care options. Using its extensive database about the problems each beneficiary is treated for each year, HCFA should be able to develop a more equitable method for paying managed care plans for providing care to Medicare beneficiaries. In this way, the cost of the Medicare + Choice options should be more comparable to the cost of providing care under traditional Medicare even if the traditional system is subject to adverse selection based on beneficiaries' health status.

Increase Premiums Paid by Beneficiaries for Medicare Part B Coverage
As discussed in Chapter 5, Part B of Medicare is optional for eligible seniors. Those who elect to sign up for Part B pay a monthly premium for this added coverage. The federal government automatically deducts the premium from the Social Security check of the beneficiary. Nearly all Medicare beneficiaries sign up for Part B coverage.

When Medicare was first established in the 1960s the funds received from the Part B premiums were intended to pay for 50% of the cost of providing Part B services. In the face of rapidly rising costs Congress quickly backtracked on this initial policy goal and allowed the share of the cost covered by premiums to fall well below this level. By the 1990s Part B premiums accounted for less than 25% of the cost of services. The Balanced Budget Act mandated that Part B premiums would be set at a level that would pay 25% of Part B costs. This initial rise meant an increase in monthly premiums of all seniors covered under Part B. In addition, as Part B costs rise in the future (as they are projected to do), the monthly premium each senior pays will also rise.

Reduce Payments to Physicians The Balanced Budget Act also mandated that its payments to physicians under fee-for-service Medicare would be reduced. It did this by reducing the amount it would pay for each service covered under the resource-based relative value scale (RBRVS) payment method. (See Chapter 5 for a discussion of RBRVS.) It also created a formula under which any increases in RBRVS payment in the future would be reduced if it can be demonstrated that physicians in aggregate are charging more for the same services through a practice referred to as "up-coding." The RBRVS system assigns a certain number of resource units to each procedure. A procedure that is more involved or more complex will be assigned more units than one that is less so. There has been evidence to suggest that, in response to relatively low rates of payment per unit, physicians reclassify the care they provide as being more complex than the service they actually provided. A more complex service generally has a higher code number and is associated with a higher number of resource units. Thus redefining the complexity of a service so as to obtain a higher level of payment is "up-coding."

Reduce in Payments to Teaching Hospitals As also discussed in Chapter 5, Medicare reimburses teaching hospitals most of the cost of training resident physicians. The Balanced Budget Act reduces the amount paid to teaching hospitals for this training, caps the number of residents that can be trained, and provides financial incentives for hospitals to decrease the number of residents in their programs.

The Best-Laid Plans... : Unintended Consequences of the Balanced Budget Act

The Balanced Budget Act of 1997 was intended to stabilize the financing of the Medicare program while maintaining the quality and accessibility of care to beneficiaries. As is often the case with complex policy changes, the act has failed to achieve many of its intended outcomes. In some cases, the results of the policy changes have been the opposite of what was intended, as described below.

Decreased Availability and Increased Cost for Medicare HMOs

The federal government had data to show that many Medicare HMOs were being paid more than was intended, due to favorable selection of enrolled beneficiaries. The reduced capitation rate included in the Balanced Budget Act was intended to rectify this imbalance. The intent was that HMOs and other managed care plans made available through Medicare + Choice would at least maintain their coverage if not actually expand it.

Instead, many HMOs reacted to the decrease in capitation payment by simply canceling their risk contract with HCFA, and in doing so canceling the HMO coverage of beneficiaries previously covered in their plan. HMOs have the option of canceling contracts on a county-by-county basis. Since the capitation rates were set on a countywide basis, the rates in one county could be quite different than the rates in nearby counties. Thus HMOs are allowed to "disenroll" covered beneficiaries in one county while maintaining coverage in others. In 1999 and 2000, the two years following enactment of the Balanced Budget Act, HMOs pulled out of more than 400 counties in 33 states, leading to the involuntary disenrollment of more than 700,000 Medicare beneficiaries. In 2001 more than 933,000 additional beneficiaries were to be involuntarily disenrolled. The reason given by most HMOs for canceling their Medicare contracts was low payment rates. In attempting to adjust capitation rates to a more equitable level, the Balanced Budget Act has led to a mass exodus of HMOs from Medicare, affecting more than 25% of those beneficiaries enrolled in HMOs. Some beneficiaries who lost their coverage were able to switch into other HMOs. Many did not have this option and were required to revert to traditional Medicare coverage. For those seniors with chronic medical problems who had to revert to traditional coverage, finding a private medigap insurer to supplement Medicare coverage often proved difficult. Those seniors who were able to maintain HMO coverage are facing dramatic increases in premiums, often as high as 200–300%. In addition, they are finding that the extra benefits previously offered by HMOs are being substantially reduced. Especially vulnerable to reductions in coverage are prescription drugs. Many seniors who joined HMOs principally to obtain prescription drug coverage now find this coverage markedly reduced.

The exodus of HMOs from the Medicare market and the distrust this change created among Medicare beneficiaries dealt a severe blow to the very concept of Medicare + Choice. Intended by its congressional sponsors to expand the range of market-based options available to seniors, few non-HMO managed care plans have elected to open their enrollment to Medicare beneficiaries. Intended as a means to privatize large parts of the

Medicare program, instead the Medicare + Choice provisions included in the Balanced Budget Act remain largely untested.

Little Interest in Medical Savings Accounts

As described above, the Balanced Budget Act made medical savings accounts (MSAs) available to seniors on a trial basis. Congress also acted to make MSAs available to employees of small businesses. Both the Medicare MSA program and the small-business MSA program were to be on a trial basis, with further analysis done to determine if they should be expanded to the general public. Unfortunately, few insurance companies, few Medicare beneficiaries, and few small-business employees have found this option to be attractive. MSA enrollment is less than 20% of what had been hoped for. It will be difficult to achieve a reliable assessment of the wisdom and efficacy of MSAs.

Financial Hardship for Hospitals, Especially Teaching and Disproprotionate Share Hospitals

The reductions in payments to hospitals included in the Balanced Budget Act were intended primarily to stabilize the Part A Trust Fund. There was no desire on the part of Congress to cause financial hardship for hospitals. Nevertheless the reductions created substantial financial hardship for a number of hospitals. Already hit by decreasing payment rates from HMOs and other managed care plans in the general health care market, many hospitals relied on Medicare payments to maintain financial stability. The reductions in Medicare payments were more than many hospitals could withstand. Hospitals in many cities have faced either closing to prevent insolvency or selling out to larger hospital corporations. Teaching hospitals and disproportionate-share hospitals faced additional losses, leading many of them to the brink of insolvency. Perhaps hardest hit were those hospitals with the dual role of caring for the poor and training physicians. Many of these hospitals are in the inner-city and are supported by local public funds. These hospitals lost out three ways: through reduced PPS payments, through reduced teaching payments, and through reduced disproportionate-share payments. A number of hospitals in this situation have had to close down, leaving many of the most vulnerable segments of our population with even greater difficulty in obtaining care.

Fortunately Congress and HCFA quickly became aware of the unintended consequences the Balanced Budget Act had on hospitals. The Balanced Budget Refinement Act, passed in 1999, increased payments to hospitals (though not back to the level before the act) so as to maintain their financial stability.

Reduced Access to Physicians

Because of reductions in the payment they receive from Medicare for treating beneficiaries, many physicians are reexamining their decision to treat Medicare patients at all. There is growing concern that any further reductions in Medicare payments to physicians will lead to widespread problems in access to physicians of the type typical of the Medicaid program.

Concept 8.5

The Balanced Budget Act of 1997 had a number of adverse consequences that Congress had not intended. Among these were a large-scale exodus of many HMOs from the Medicare program and severe financial hardship for many hospitals.

Why Did Medicare HMOs Have So Little Success in Holding Down Costs?

The rising cost of health care seen generally in this country over the past 30 years led to rising costs for Medicare as well. The federal government took a number of steps that were very successful in constraining that rise. Examples of these successful policy changes include the PPS system and the RBRVS method of paying physicians.

The move to managed care as an alternative to fee-for-service has been substantially less successful. Initially, enrollment in Medicare HMOs grew rapidly. However, when it was discovered that Medicare HMOs were benefiting substantially from favorable selection of enrollees, Congress acted to reduce payments to HMOs to a more equitable level. At the same time Congress took a number of other steps intended both to stabilize the long-term finances of Medicare and to shift the program to a more market-based plan.

The privatization of Medicare has turned out to be largely a failure, at least to date. Rather than reducing costs, it actually increased costs, and subsequently has resulted in the abrupt, involuntary disenrollment of more than one-quarter of all covered beneficiaries.

Why have HMOs and other managed care plans not turned out to save money compared to fee-for-service alternatives? As noted in Chapter 4, the original Rand Health Insurance Experiment carried out in the 1980s demonstrated that HMOs saved money over their fee-for-service competitors largely in the way they used the hospital. HMO patients were hospitalized less often and for shorter periods. Now recall that the Medicare PPS system, also enacted in the 1980s, was quite successful in reducing hospital costs for Medicare beneficiaries. It may be that the PPS system had achieved roughly the same savings in hospital costs for Medicare beneficiaries that HMOs had achieved for the general public. There may not have been any further savings to be realized by switching Medicare from a fee-for-service to a capitated system of payment. Once again HCFA, Congress, and presidential candidates must contend with a Medicare program that sits on unstable ground—a program that may face added instability once the baby-boom generation starts filing for Medicare eligibility in the next 10–15 years.

ON-LINE DATA SOURCES

Most of the data used in this chapter come from documents that are publicly
  available on the Internet. Some of the most important sites are listed below,
  with examples of useful reports available through these sites. Readers are
  encouraged to search these sites for additional information on recent and current
  changes to the Medicare program.
U.S. Health Care Financing Administration: www.hcfa.gov
  Balanced Budget Act of 1997—Medicare and Medicaid Provisions, 1998
  Protecting Medicare Beneficiaries After Medicare+Choice Organizations Withdraw, June 2000
  Medicare and Managed Care web page:
    www.hcfa.gov/medicare/mgdcar1.htm
U.S. General Accounting Office: www.gao.gov
  Medicare Managed Care Plans: Many Factors Contribute to Recent Withdrawals; Plan Interest Continues. GAO/HEHS-99-91, April 1999
  Medicare: Progress to Date in Implementing Certain Major Balanced Budget Act Reforms. GAO/T-HEHS-99-87, March 17, 1999
  Medicare+Choice: Impact of 1997 Balanced Budget Act Payment Reforms on Beneficiaries and Plans. GAO/T-HEHS-99-137, June 9, 1999
Kaiser Family Foundation: www.kff.org
  Medicare+Choice Overview. July 1998
  Medicare Managed Care Overview. September 1999
  How Medicare HMO Withdrawals Affect Beneficiary Benefits, Costs, and Continuity of Care. November 1999

CHAPTER 9

Long-Term Care

Key Concepts

- The very population group that is most in need of long-term care—those over 85 years old—is also the fastest growing population group in the United States.

- Medicare pays very little of the national cost of nursing home care—about 12% in 1997. Patients who need long-term, custodial nursing home care are not eligible for Medicare payment.

- Medicaid will pay the cost of long-term, custodial nursing care for those seniors who need it. However, before becoming eligible for Medicaid payment, seniors must first exhaust

nearly all their own resources by paying for care out of pocket.

- Medicare has become the principal source of payment for home health services for the elderly and disabled. Following a relaxation in eligibility guidelines in the 1980s, both the number of visits per home care patient and overall program costs have increased dramatically.

- Hospice care has become an increasingly important source of care for patients with terminal illness. Hospice care involves treating symptoms rather than prolonging life, as well as offering emotional support for dying patients and their family.

U p to this point this book has talked mostly about the system of acute care in the United States. Most of the money spent on health care, and most of the attention given to recent changes in the market for health care, have focused on the care we provide to people with specific conditions that need the care of a physician or a hospital.

What happens, though, when elderly or disabled people are not sick enough to require hospitalization but, due to chronic illness or general frailty, are not able to take care of themselves? In such cases, assistance is provided through our system of long-term care. As the name implies, this type of care is ongoing, and has less to do with the treatment of a specific disease until it is cured than with care for chronic conditions for which there is no cure.

There are many reasons for people to need long-term care. Most often the elderly patient simply has physical difficulty undertaking normal daily activities such as dressing, bathing, eating, and going to the toilet. (Such activities are referred to as "activities of daily living" or ADLs.) Alternatively a patient may have a serious mental impairment such as Alzheimer's disease that necessitates continuous supervision. Some patients may have both physical difficulty with ADLs and mental impairment.

Traditionally the need for long-term care has been met principally by the family. As people became frail and in need of assistance, younger family members often team together to provide care. However, as the American family has changed over the years, more and more frail elderly patients need organized institutions or services to help them. In 1982, 74% of people in need of long-term care were cared for in their home by family members or friends. By 1994 this number had been reduced to 64% (Liu et al. 2000).

The Growing Need for Long-Term Care Among the Frail Elderly

Most people over 65 years old are able to care for themselves without any need for long-term care services. The problem of long-term care is mainly a problem of the frail elderly. It is the very old—those over 85—who typically need long-term care. Of the 35 million people over the age of 65 in the United States in 2000, about 12% were over 85 (data from the U.S. Census Bureau). However, half of all people in nursing homes and one-quarter of all people with long term care needs living in the community were over 85. As Figure 9.1 shows, the number of people over 85 is growing much more rapidly than the number of elderly overall.

In 2000 there were 4.3 million people in this country who were 85 years or older. By 2020 this number is projected to increase to 6.8 million; by 2040 the number will be 14.3 million. As a result of the baby-boom generation moving into their elder years, those over 85 will grow from 12% of the elderly population in 2000 to 19% by 2040. Whatever problems our health care system has in providing and financing long-term care will be multiplied within a few decades.

Concept 9.1

The very population group that is most in need of long-term care—those over 85 years old—is also the fastest growing population group in the United States.

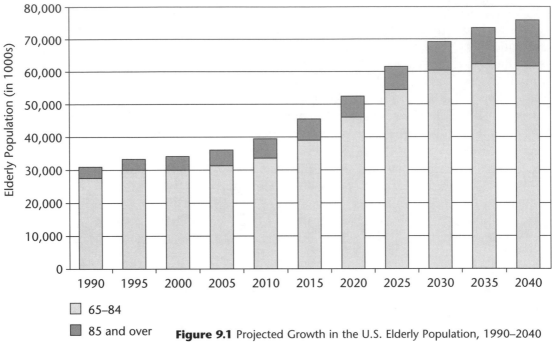

Figure 9.1 Projected Growth in the U.S. Elderly Population, 1990–2040
Source: U.S. Census Bureau

Nursing Home Care

If an elderly or disabled person is in need of long-term care that, for whatever reason, cannot be provided in the home, that person can receive care in a nursing home or other type of residential care facility. At any one time about 5% of the elderly, or about 1.75 million people, are receiving long-term care in some sort of a nursing facility.

The average age of people in nursing homes is about 84. Seventy-two percent are women. Eighty-three percent of these residents needed assistance with at least three ADLs; 70% had severe memory loss (data from the Kaiser Family Foundation).

Not all people in nursing homes, however, are there for chronic long-term care. Many people will spend a short time in a nursing home following an acute illness or injury, but will return home after a short stay. As many as one in five elderly people will spend at least some time in a nursing home at some point during their life. Although the average length of stay for those in nursing homes is about 15 months, 50% of patients stay less than one month. About 20% of nursing home patients stay there for two years or more.

Many people have the impression that Medicare pays for most of the nursing home care needed by the elderly. As Figure 9.2 illustrates, this is usually not the case.

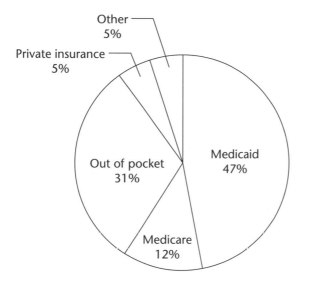

Figure 9.2 Who Pays for Nursing Home Care
Source: HCFA, for 1997

Other — 5%

Private insurance — 5%

Out of pocket 31%

Medicaid 47%

Medicare 12%

Medicare pays for about 12% of nursing home care. In order to qualify for Medicare payment, a patient must have an acute medical problem that requires skilled nursing care as part of the treatment program. Examples of *skilled nursing care* would be the administration of intravenous antibiotics or assistance with rehabilitation following surgery or a stroke. In each case a physician must certify that skilled care of this type is medically indicated. In most cases the patient must have been in an acute care hospital just prior to entering the nursing home to qualify for Medicare payment. Even when a patient qualifies for skilled nursing care of this type, Medicare will pay the full cost only for the first 20 days. For skilled nursing care required beyond 20 days the patient must make $97 per day copayment up to a maximum of 100 days of care. Any care required after 100 days is totally the responsibility of the patient, with no further coverage from Medicare.

Medicare distinguishes between skilled nursing care and custodial nursing care. Once a patient's medical condition has plateaued—that is, once he has attained the maximum level of healing or rehabilitation that can be expected in the short term—the patient no longer qualifies for Medicare's skilled nursing benefit. If he has to remain in the nursing home due to his need for assistance with ADLs, he is now considered to be receiving *custodial care* rather than skilled nursing care. Medicare does not pay for custodial care in nursing homes. Patients who need this type of care must find another way to pay for that care.

One of the advantages of Medicare's HMO option has been a relaxation in Medicare policies pertaining to the use of skilled nursing facilities. Doctors in a Medicare HMO are allowed to treat a patient in a skilled nursing facility at their discretion. The patient need not have been in a hospital first. The cost of skilled nursing care comes out of the overall yearly capitation received by the HMO, which typically places some type of utilization control on the use of long-term care. The type of control depends on the type of HMO, but it often involves a case manager—a nurse who supervises the overall process of care a frail elderly patient will receive. However, the patient still must require skilled nursing care to be eligible for nursing home payment under Medicare HMOs. If the patient needs ongoing custodial care, Medicare HMOs, like traditional Medicare, provide no coverage.

Concept 9.2

Medicare pays very little of the national cost of nursing home care—about 12% in 1997. Patients who need long-term, custodial nursing home care are not eligible for Medicare payment.

What does the patient do, then, who no longer needs skilled nursing care but still needs constant assistance with ADLs? Consider the case, for example, of an elderly widow who has been living alone in her own home, but who suffers a stroke and is partially paralyzed. Medicare will pay the costs of a short-term rehabilitation program, but after a few weeks the patient is no longer eligible for coverage. Returning home is not a realistic option, so the patient finds herself in a nursing home. The cost of that nursing home will typically be between $45,000 and $55,000 per year. Who pays for the ongoing care this patient needs? There are three principal sources to pay for this care, described below.

1. Pay for Nursing Home Care Out-of-Pocket

Many patients find themselves with no way to pay for nursing home care other than to pay out of pocket. In 1997, patients and their families paid 31% of the cost of nursing home care out of personal resources. Of those patients admitted to nursing homes, about one in four pays for care out of pocket. At $50,000 a year or more, it doesn't take long to exhaust the patient's resources. Few seniors have sufficient assets to be able to generate an income of $50,000 a year on an on going basis. Nonetheless, in many cases there is no alternative for the patient but to exhaust her personal assets in paying for care.

2. Medicaid Payment for Nursing Home Care

Unlike Medicare, the Medicaid program will pay the costs of ongoing, custodial care in nursing homes for poor seniors. Recall from Chapter 6 that nearly three-fourths of Medicaid funds go to pay for the care of elderly and disabled people who are also poor. Elderly, poor people who need long-term care in a nursing home or other type of custodial care facility are eligible to have Medicaid pay the full cost of their care. This is our country's final safety net to ensure that no elderly or disabled person who needs custodial nursing care will be denied that care because he or she is unable to pay for it. About two-thirds of long-term nursing home residents nationwide are covered by Medicaid.

An irony of our system of paying for nursing home care is the extent to which it causes people who were not originally poor to become poor. As described above, about one nursing home patient in four who needs ongoing custodial care will pay for that care out of pocket. For many of these people it takes very little time to completely exhaust one's life savings paying for nursing home care. Once a patient spends all (or at least nearly all) of his money paying for nursing home care, he then becomes eligible for Medicaid payment for any further care. He is allowed to keep up to $2000 in a personal savings account, but otherwise must sell all assets and use all the funds before Medicaid will pay for his care. Of those patients who initially pay for their nursing home care out of pocket and end up staying in the nursing home for two or three years or more, half will become impoverished and become eligible for Medicaid payment for their care.

> ## *Concept 9.3*
>
> Medicaid will pay the cost of long-term, custodial nursing care for those seniors who need it. However, before becoming eligible for Medicaid payment, seniors must first exhaust nearly all their own resources by paying for care out of pocket.

What happens in the case of an elderly couple who have been living in their own home for years and one spouse sustains an illness or injury that requires long-term, custodial care in a nursing home? The spouse in the nursing home requires ongoing care, yet the healthy spouse is still able to stay at home and live independently. Historically this couple was required to spend all their money, including exhausting their combined savings *and* selling their house and using the proceeds, to pay for the nursing home care of the ill spouse. It was necessary for both spouses to become impoverished for Medicaid to cover the care of the ill spouse. The spouse remaining in the home faced a heart-wrenching choice: either spend all your money, lose your home, and become poor, or divorce your spouse and sever legal responsibility for the cost of his nursing home care. For years the need to protect the financial independence of the healthy spouse was a major contributor to the rate of divorce among elderly couples, many of whom had been married for decades.

Fortunately Congress changed the rules on what has come to be called "Medicaid spend-down." Now if a couple faces the need to have one spouse cared for in a nursing home, the other spouse is allowed to maintain assets sufficient to remain in the home and live independently.

What if an elderly person with substantial personal assets finds that she needs to be in a nursing home? Why not simply give all her money to her children, thus becoming poor and qualifying for Medicaid? When Congress changed the law to protect the remaining spouse from Medicaid spend-down, it also changed the law regarding giving away one's assets. There is now a "look-back" period, typically about three years, in which Medicaid can look to see if the patient gave away significant assets to children or other family members. If it is found that she did give away assets that she otherwise would have been required to spend before qualifying for Medicaid, the family members who received the gifts must first use those funds to pay for the needed nursing home care. Only after the gifted funds have been used will the patient qualify for Medicaid coverage for her long-term care needs.

3. Private Long-Term Care Insurance

A number of private insurance companies are looking at the option of offering insurance specifically to cover the cost of long-term care. These types of policies are usually made available to large employee groups. Only those not currently in need of long-term care are eligible to obtain the policies. The cost of these policies can be prohibitive—over $2,500 per year for someone who is 65 years old and over $7,500 per year for someone 75 years old. As a result few individuals can afford such coverage. About 7% of the elderly population is covered by private long-term care insurance, and 5% of the cost of nursing home care is paid by these policies.

Home Health Care

A substantial number of elderly or disabled people in this country need help with ADLs on an ongoing basis but are not so ill that they need to be in a nursing home. If they are provided with a limited amount of assistance these people are capable of remaining in their home. Many of them qualify for in-home, long-term care under both Medicare and Medicaid.

Typically people who qualify for home care assistance have a nurse visit them on a regular basis, checking on their situation and ensuring that their basic needs are met. These nurses can provide services such as monitoring the patient's medications, assessing the patient's nutrition, and evaluating ongoing home safety. In addition some of these patients may be eligible to have the assistance of a home health aide. An aide of this type is not a nurse but rather someone trained specifically in providing assistance with ADLs. The aide will visit the patient on a regular basis and help with such activities as bathing and meal preparation.

Medicare is the principal source of payment for long-term home health services. This is in sharp contrast to nursing home care, in which Medicaid is the principal payer for long-term services. In 1997 Medicare spent $16.7 billion on home health care and the Medicaid program, covering both elderly and nonelderly people in need of home health care, spent $6.6 billion (data from HCFA).

The Medicare home health benefit was originally intended to be similar to the nursing home benefit: it would only cover a short period of care and only after hospitalization for an acute medical problem. In the 1980s Congress modified the eligibility rules in two important ways:

- It removed the requirement that the patient must be in the hospital before being eligible for home care services.
- It removed the cap on the number of services an eligible patient may receive per year.

Now any Medicare beneficiary who meets the following criteria is eligible for payment for home health services on an ongoing basis. If patients meet all these criteria, they are eligible to have Medicare pay for both the skilled care services and the custodial care services provided in the home.

- The patient is homebound.
- The patient is under the care of a physician, who periodically reviews the plan for home care services.
- The patient has an intermittent need for skilled care services from either a nurse or other care provider (e.g., physical therapist).
- Care is provided by a home health agency that is a certified provider of services under the Medicare program.

Figure 9.3 shows the increase in the cost of home health services covered by Medicare between 1974 and 1997. It can be seen that costs began to increase around 1980, when some of the initial program restrictions were relaxed. In 1989 there was a further loosening of eligibility requirements, and the costs of the program began to soar. In the nine years from

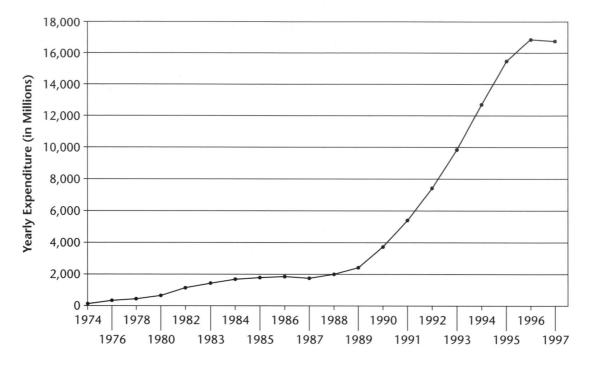

Figure 9.3 Yearly Medicare Expenditures for Home Health Services, 1974–1997
Source: HCFA

1980 to 1989 the cost of the program nearly tripled, from $662 million to $2.25 billion. In the years from 1989–1997 they increased nearly ninefold, to $16.7 billion.

Figure 9.4 shows the change in the frequency with which home care services were used over this same time period. For most of the period from 1974–1989, those beneficiaries who qualified for Medicare home health services received about 25 visits per year. With the relaxation of eligibility requirements in the late 1980s, the average number of visits per home health care beneficiary jumped to nearly 75 per year.

Concept 9.4

Medicare has become the principal source of payment for home health services for the elderly and disabled. Following a relaxation in eligibility guidelines in the 1980s, both the number of visits per home care patient and overall program costs have increased dramatically.

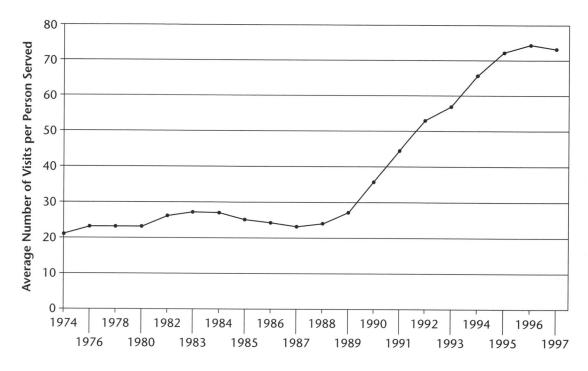

Figure 9.4 Average Number of Home Health Visits per Year, per Person Served, 1974–1997

Source: HCFA

The Medicare home health program was initially intended as a low-cost supplement to hospital care. In 1967 it accounted for less than 1% of all Medicare expenditures. Over the next 30 years it became a major service program, by 1997 accounting for nearly 10% of all Medicare expenditures. As discussed in Chapter 8, the cost of home health care originally came out of the Part A Hospital Trust Fund. As Part A costs rose and the Trust Fund was facing potential insolvency, Congress modified Medicare's home health program in 1997 as part of the Balanced Budget Act. It reallocated most of the costs of the program to Medicare Part B, and instituted new limitations on the use of home health services. Preliminary indications are that these changes in eligibility and payment were successful in reducing costs, with a 12.9% decline in expenditures between 1997 and 1998. The effect these changes will have on the beneficiaries receiving home health services and their ability to remain in their homes remains to be determined.

Medicaid and Home Health Care

Although Medicare is the principal payer for home health services, the Medicaid program also plays an important role. In 1997, 1.9 million people were eligible for home health care under Medicaid. Of elderly adults in need of home health services, 19% are covered by Medicaid as well as Medicare. Of adults under 65 who need home health services, 25% are covered by Medicaid and an additional 12% are covered by both Medicaid and Medicare. If one looks only at poor adults under 65 who need home health care, 64% are covered by Medicaid (data from Kaiser Family Foundation).

Hospice Care

Consider the case of an elderly patient who discovers that he has cancer or some other terminal illness and is told by his doctor that he will most likely die within the next six months. Often this type of patient either is not sick enough to be in the hospital, or alternatively simply doesn't want to be in the hospital due to the futility of future attempts at treatment. It can be very difficult for the family by itself to provide adequate care to a dying person, yet neither the patient nor his family want him to be in a nursing home. For this patient, a hospice may provide the best care available.

A hospice can be either a place for a person with a terminal disease to go for treatment, a team of professionals who assist the family in providing care to the terminally ill in the home, or both. The hospice program focuses on relieving suffering rather than prolonging life. Hospice care involves a shift in the emphasis of care away from further attempts at cure to controlling the symptoms of the illness and providing emotional support during the dying process. Emotional support is offered both to the patient and to his family members. Hospice care begins at the point that the inevitability of death is recognized and carries beyond the patient's death to help family members adjust to the loss.

The modern hospice movement, with an emphasis on symptom control and on dying as a process, began in England in the 1960s. The first modern hospice was named St. Christopher's, and is described in the following quotation.

> Several factors differentiate St. Christopher's from hospitals: allowing children to visit and play, personalized care, little patient-staff protocol, an informal social life, a continuum of care including home care, freedom to issue drugs and liquor as requested for symptom control, and follow-up with the family members after the patient's death. (Plumb and Ogle 1992)

As it has developed in the United States over the past 30 years, a hospice program usually involves a health care team, often including a physician, a nurse, a social worker, a member of the clergy, trained home health aides, and community volunteers. Team members come to the patient's home and provide as much care there as feasible. They often provide respite care to relieve the family for periods of time so they can take a break from the intense responsibilities of caring for a dying person. Some hospice programs also have a care center, typical to that described for St. Christopher's. The patient who needs intensive assistance can stay in the facility, with family members visiting freely. Alternatively the patient can split his time, spending part of the week in the hospice facility and part of the week at home with family members. As one might expect, hospice patients are three times as likely to die at home rather than in a hospital or nursing home when compared to comparable patients who do not use hospice services.

Congress amended the Medicare program in 1982 to allow payment for hospice services for beneficiaries. In order to be eligible for hospice care,

- The beneficiary must be certified by his physician to be suffering from an incurable disease and expected to live six months or less

- The beneficiary must also agree to waive Medicare coverage for treatment of his illness provided outside the hospice program.

Thus a hospice patient under Medicare agrees to forgo further surgery or other types of therapy that are not intended for palliation and symptom relief. In return the beneficiary is eligible for a substantially wider range of services than is available under traditional Medicare, such as drugs required for symptom relief, respite care at an inpatient facility, and bereavement counseling for the family.

The number of Medicare beneficiaries choosing to use hospice programs increased substantially during the 1990s, from 143,000 in 1992 to nearly 360,000 in 1998. During this same period the number of hospice programs providing care grew from 1208 in 1992 to 2281 in 1998 (data from the United States General Accounting Office).

As the use of hospice programs and facilities expanded, the type of patient using hospice care changed somewhat. In 1992, 76% of all hospice patients were eligible for services because of a diagnosis of cancer. In 1998 this number had decreased to 57%. An increasing number of patients with diseases such as heart disease, lung disease, stroke, or Alzheimer's disease had entered hospice programs. Despite this relative decline nearly half of all Medicare patients who died of cancer were enrolled in a hospice program at the time of their death.

Although Medicare beneficiaries are eligible for a full six months of hospice care, the actual length of time in a hospice program before death is usually considerably shorter. In 1992 the median length of hospice service was 26 days (mean 74 days). In 1998 the median had decreased to 19 days (mean 59 days). This means that half of all hospice patients in 1998 received fewer than three weeks of service. These data suggest that it is still difficult for physicians, patients, and family members to face the inevitability of death that confronts many patients, and to begin to plan for death in advance of the final stages of illness.

Concept 9.5

Hospice care has become an increasingly important source of care for patients with terminal illness. Hospice care involves treating symptoms rather than prolonging life, as well as offering emotional support for dying patients and their families.

Life-Care Communities as an Alternative to Long-Term Care

The options for long-term care have expanded recently with the addition of a relatively new type of senior care facility—the life-care community. A life-care community offers a permanent place for seniors to live in which their needs for assistance with living will be taken care of, no matter how long they need them. Whatever level of services a resident needs will be provided for one fixed cost.

A life-care community typically has several levels of care available.

1. *Independent living.* The life-care community provides individual apartments or condominiums for those residents capable of living alone. The resident in this level of care is fully independent, providing her own meals, and not relying on assistance for any activities of daily living. She may, however, obtain meals from a central dining facility when desired, have assistance with transportation, and have someone always available for assistance in case of an emergency.

2. *Assisted living.* Some residents are not fully capable of living independently, but are not frail enough to require constant assistance. Typically the life-care facility provides this resident with an apartment in a central facility that has staff immediately available. These residents can make the apartment their own home. They usually require little if any help with ADLs, although they may eat in a central dining room and may have assistance managing their medications and bathing. The apartments usually have call buttons and other surveillance devices, so if a resident ever needs assistance, it will be immediately available. These facilities are staffed around the clock, usually with aides rather than nurses.

3. *Custodial care.* Residents in life-care communities sometimes suffer an illness or injury that necessitates round-the-clock assistance with ADLs or

medical needs. This is the level of care that is usually provided in a nursing home. The life-care facility has a fully staffed nursing facility available for these residents. The resident may need this level of care for only a short period, after which he can move back to his own home or apartment, or he may need this care for the rest of his life, in which case he will remain in the nursing center.

The unique aspect of life-care communities is that all these services are available for one fixed fee. The fee usually involves both a cash buy-in when the resident first enters the community, and a monthly maintenance fee. In return for the buy-in and the monthly fee, the resident is guaranteed whatever level of care she needs, for the rest of her life. The only requirements are that the resident demonstrate sufficient income to ensure lifetime payment of the maintenance fees, and that she enter the community at level 1 (i.e., she initially is healthy enough to live independently).

Life-care communities offer an attractive alternative to many seniors who face the prospect of growing old alone at home and possibly ending their life in a nursing home. However, for a life-care community to work, the senior must plan for her remaining years when she is still relatively healthy. If she waits until she needs extensive assistance, she is no longer eligible to enter these communities.

As one might imagine, it can often be very expensive to enter a life-care community, making them realistic alternatives for only the wealthiest seniors. However, a number of religious and other nonprofit institutions have established life-care communities, making them available to people without a large number of assets. Whether they will become a major source of long-term care remains to be seen.

Future Policy Issues in Long-Term Care

A number of policy questions remain to be answered regarding the future of long-term care in the United States. As difficult as the problems of the health care system in general are, the problems confronting our long-term care system are often even more vexing, and are complicated by the relative lack of attention long-term care receives in the public health policy arena.

How Will We Provide Long-Term Care for the Growing Number of Frail Elderly?

As discussed above, the number of people in this country over 85, the population most in need of long-term care services, is expected to more than triple in the next 40 years, growing from 12% of the overall elderly population to 19%. Many of these people will need nursing home care. Many states have placed limits on the construction of new nursing home beds, leading to an 18% nationwide decline between 1974 and 1994 in the number of beds per 1000 people over 85. How will we build the nursing home facilities to meet the growing future need?

An alternative to building more nursing home beds is to develop more community-based services. In many cases a well-designed program of home health services can allow patients in need of substantial assistance to remain in the home with their families. For those without families to help them, smaller, community-based residential facilities that provide a more home-like atmosphere can be an attractive alternative to traditional nursing homes.

How Will We Pay for Long-Term Care in the Future?

More challenging than simply building the facilities needed for care is the question of how we will pay for that care. Few will argue that the current system of financing long-term care is optimal. Many question whether the impoverishment of elderly, middle-class nursing home residents is a wise choice. Is the best option to ask people to pay for nursing home care out of pocket? Similarly, is the way we split responsibility between Medicaid and Medicare wise, with Medicaid paying for nursing home care and Medicare paying for home health care?

Long-term care can be seen as a broad social need that needs to be addressed through broad social policy means. A system of social insurance, similar to the Medicare system of paying for acute care, could potentially meet the financing needs for long-term care. In order to do so, however, it will need to be broadly financed by all taxpayers, not just those who need care. The American taxpayer has been especially reluctant in recent years to take on new social programs. Yet, a substantial portion of the financing burden of long-term care falls on middle-class families and individuals. Will the American taxpayer be willing to invest in long-term care now so that needed care is available in the coming decades?

How Will We Maintain the Quality of the Long-Term Care System?

For years there has been concern over the quality of long-term care services, especially care in nursing homes. As many as one nursing home in four has been found to have ongoing quality problems (Feder et al. 2000). Issues such as the appropriate level of staffing, the use of physical and chemical restraints, and the quality of the nursing services provided have led to continued federal and state oversight.

One of the issues contributing to these problems has been the relatively low level of Medicaid payment for nursing home care. As with acute medical care, Medicaid pays providers substantially less for nursing home care than private payment sources. With the large number of Medicaid beneficiaries in nursing homes it has often been difficult for providers both to meet quality requirements and to maintain financial viability. The trade-off between cost and quality will remain an important issue in long-term care.

Who Will Provide the Medical Care for the Frail Elderly?

Quality long-term care requires the continuous participation and oversight of medical personnel. However, a number of physicians are either unwilling or unable to provide active supervision of long-term care. Recent years have seen a resurgence in interest in primary care among physicians. If the growing needs of the elderly are to be met, that interest in primary care will need to expand to include additional emphasis on geriatric care. This can be done either by including more involvement in geriatric care in the training of general internists and family physicians, or increasing the number of physicians who focus their practice on geriatric care. As an alternative, nurse practitioners and other types of midlevel health care practitioners can assume a greater role in monitoring and supervising long-term care.

What Are the Ethical Issues Surrounding the Care of the Frail Elderly?

In recent years there has been increased attention to important ethical aspects of long-term care. The increasing role of advance directives, such as living-wills and durable power of attorney, has provided the opportunity for many elderly persons to consider the level of care they wish to receive in the event that they become seriously ill. Issues of the autonomy and privacy of residents of nursing homes, especially those with cognitive impairment, are only beginning to be examined. The question of physician-assisted suicide has begun to receive increased attention as an option for patients facing inevitable death combined with intractable suffering. Future policy discussions need to include consideration of these and other ethical issues that surround long-term care.

REFERENCES AND ON-LINE DATA SOURES

Feder J, Komisar HL, Niefeld M. Long-Term Care in the United States: An Overview. *Health Affairs* 2000 19(3):40–56.

Kaiser Family Foundation. Long-Term Care: Medicaid's Role and Challenges. November, 1999, available at www.kff.org/content/2000/2172/.

Liu K, Manton KG, Aragon C. Changes in Home Care Use by Older People with Disabilities: 1982–1994 —Executive Summary. Washington, DC: AARP Public

Policy Institute, January 2000, available at
www.research.aarp.org/health/2000_02_homecare_1.html.

U.S. General Accounting Office. Long-Term Care—Baby Boom Generation
Presents Financing Challenges. March 9, 1998, GAO/T-HEHS-98-107,
available at www.access.gpo.gov/su_docs/aces/aces160.shtml.

Current data and projections about future population statistics are available from
the U.S. Census Bureau at www.census.gov/.

HCFA data on nursing home expenditures are available from the following sources:
www.hcfa.gov/stats/NHE-OAct/

U.S. Health Care Financing Administration. Medicare and Medicaid Statistical
Supplement, 1999. *Health Care Financing Review*, 1999.

Levit K, Cowan C, Lazenby H, et al. (U.S. Health Care Financing Administration).
Health Spending in 1998: Signals of Change. *Health Affairs* 2000;
19(1):124–32.

Data about hospice programs are from the following sources:

U.S. General Accounting Office. Medicare—More Beneficiaries Use Hospice But
for Fewer Days of Care. September 2000, GAO/HEHS-00-182, available at
www.access.gpo.gov/su_docs/aces/aces160.shtml.

Plumb JD, Ogle KS. Hospice Care. *Primary Care; Clinics in Office Practice* 1992;
19(4):807–20.

Information and data about long-term care insurance are available in the following government report:

Long-Term Care Insurance—Better Information Critical to Prospective Purchasers.
September 13, 2000, GAO/T-HEHS-00-196, available at
www.access.gpo.gov/su_docs/aces/aces160.shtml.

CHAPTER 10

The Uninsured

Key Concepts

- At the beginning of World War II in 1941 fewer than 10 million Americans were covered by health insurance. The vast majority of the population was uninsured, paying for needed health care out of pocket.

- The problem of the uninsured is not principally a problem affecting low-income families. Nearly two-thirds of uninsured Americans are in families with annual household income above $25,000.

- The uninsured are made up mostly of young Americans. Twenty-four percent are children. Thirty-eight percent are young adults.

- Minority ethnic groups are overrepresented among the uninsured. This is especially true for Hispanics.

- Low-wage workers are offered employer-sponsored health insurance less often and accept enrollment less often than higher-wage workers. As a result of the combination of these two forces, the rate of health insurance coverage is substantially lower among low-wage workers than higher-wage workers, even though many employers make coverage available.

- Workers in small firms (fewer than 25 employees) are less than half as likely as workers in large firms (500 employees or more) to be covered by employer-sponsored health insurance.

- Requiring all employers to provide health insurance to their regular employees and their families has been demonstrated to reduce the number of uninsured substantially without imposing undue hardship on small businesses.

- As exemplified by the Children's Health Insurance Program (CHIP), national policies to extend coverage to the uninsured that rely on states to implement and carry out new insurance programs may have problems attaining program goals.

In order to gain access to most types of health services in this country, an individual or family needs to be covered by some sort of health insurance plan. The high cost of care, even relatively simple care, is often more than most people can afford to pay out of pocket. Fortunately the vast majority of Americans are covered by some type of plan that will pay for their care when needed. In 1999, 84% of Americans had health insurance coverage.

However, the remaining 16% of Americans must face the prospect of illness or injury with no health insurance, and thus no way to pay for their health care. One in six Americans is uninsured, and as a result is often unable to obtain needed care due to the cost of that care. Compared to patients with insurance, the uninsured seldom obtain the type of preventive health services that can substantially reduce rates of illness and death (Ayanian et al. 2000). Providing health care to these people poses one of the most difficult policy problems facing America today.

The United States is alone among developed countries in maintaining national policies that exclude segments of their population from health insurance coverage. Throughout the last century the United States struggled repeatedly with this issue. All indications are it will continue to struggle with it in the years to come.

The Creation and Expansion of Health Insurance in the Twentieth Century

The problem of the uninsured is a relatively recent one in American political history. For much of the twentieth century being uninsured was the norm, and was not thought to pose a serious national policy issue. Prior to the Great Depression few Americans were covered by any type of health insurance plan. Most insurance companies shied away from providing health insurance because of the difficulties in predicting or controlling the cost of care. It was the national economic crisis of the 1930s that stimulated the first widespread interest in health insurance.

Many hospitals were facing severe financial difficulties during the Great Depression, due largely to patients' inability to pay their hospital bills. The very survival of the American system of voluntary, nonprofit hospitals required some type of prepaid hospital insurance. If enough people were willing to pay a small amount each month to insure against the possible costs of a hospitalization, these funds could then be pooled to pay for the care of those who actually did get sick. Rather than relying on private insurance companies to offer this type of insurance, hospitals in most parts of the country banded together to form their own, nonprofit hospital insurance program. This was the birth of the national Blue Cross movement.

The Blue Cross insurance plans were principally intended to pay the costs of hospitalization. They did not pay for the cost of physician care. Shortly after the creation of the Blue Cross system, physicians in many areas of the country created a parallel system of nonprofit insurance for the cost of physician care: the Blue Shield program. The American Hospital Association and the American Medical Association worked together to ensure that "the Blues" (as the combined Blue Cross/Blue Shield programs were often called) remained under the local control of hospital and physician associations and out of the hands of commercial insurers.

These new insurance plans had a potential problem that could threaten their financial stability: adverse selection. Since health insurance was a relatively new option for most Americans, there was a risk that only those individuals who were actually facing illness would choose to have coverage. The success of the programs depended on spreading the cost of care over as many people as possible. If only sick people signed up for the plans, the cost of care would be more than the premiums paid by patients could support.

The solution to this problem lay in focusing on large groups of relatively healthy people as the principal market for the new health insurance. The best way to enroll large numbers of healthy people was to offer the insurance through employee groups. The concept of health insurance as an employee benefit was established through the marketing of the Blues to employee groups.

By the beginning of World War II, the idea of health insurance had caught on. Seeing the initial success of the Blues in enrolling large numbers of subscribers, private, for-profit insurance companies began to follow suit and offer plans of their own. By 1940 more than 6 million people had enrolled in the Blues, with more than 3 million people covered by some type of private health insurance. The vast majority of Americans, however, were still uninsured and paid for health care out of pocket.

Concept 10.1

At the beginning of World War II in 1941 fewer than 10 million Americans were covered by health insurance. The vast majority of the population was uninsured, paying for needed health care out of pocket.

Chapter 4 describes the two major policy decisions enacted by the federal government that led over time to employer-provided health insurance becoming the norm rather than the exception:

- The federal government exempted employer-paid fringe benefits from the national wage and price controls that were imposed during World War II.

- The federal government decided that fringe benefits obtained through work are not taxable as income to the worker.

These two policy decisions created powerful economic incentives for the expansion of employer-sponsored health plans. As labor unions bargained for improved wages and benefits for workers, one of the first benefits they sought was health insurance. By the 1960s most large companies routinely offered health insurance to their full-time workers. Health insurance became the norm for most Americans.

The 1960s saw two major shifts in health care policy: the expansion of health insurance to the poor and elderly through the Medicaid and Medicare programs, and the beginning of the rapid escalation in health care costs. By 1970 the cost of health care began to rise more rapidly than the national economy, and continued to do so for the next 25 years. In 1970 the average per capita cost of health care for all Americans was $297. By 1993, the year of the debate over President Clinton's proposed health care reforms, this figure had increased by a factor of 10 to $2937 per capita. (These data are from HCFA, and are not adjusted for inflation.) As the cost of health care rose relentlessly throughout the 1970s and 1980s, more and more people at the economic margins of American society found it difficult if not impossible to find or maintain health insurance for themselves and their families. By 1980 more than 31 million people lacked health insurance.

The Issue of the Uninsured Finds the American Mainstream: Wofford Versus Thornburgh, 1991

Until 1991 there was relatively little emphasis in either the public policy arena or the national media on how many Americans did or did not have health insurance. This situation changed dramatically following the upset victory of Harris Wofford over Richard Thornburgh in the 1991 Pennsylvania election for U.S. senator. Wofford had been appointed on an interim basis to fill an empty Senate seat. A special election had been called for November 5, 1991, to fill the seat on a permanent basis. Wofford, a Democrat, had been a cofounder of the Peace Corps and former state labor secretary, but was relatively unknown in either Pennsylvania or national politics. His Republican opponent was Richard Thornburgh, who had been governor of Pennsylvania from 1979 to 1987 and attorney general in the Bush administration. Wofford had been given little chance of beating Thornburgh. At one point he trailed Thornburgh by 40 points in preelection polls.

Wofford made a strategic decision that was to have far-reaching national implications. He began to focus his campaign on the plight of the uninsured and the need for national health insurance. This message struck a chord with Pennsylvania voters, and Wofford rapidly gained ground on Thornburgh. On election-day Wofford defeated Thornburgh by a margin of 10 percentage points. By focusing the public spotlight on the uninsured, Wofford had not only beaten one of the strongest contenders in the Republican party, he had set the stage for Bill Clinton's proposal for national health care reform and the changes that followed it, as discussed in Chapter 7.

Understanding the Uninsured: Who Are They, and Why Are They Uninsured?

The successive victories by Harris Wofford and Bill Clinton placed the problem of the uninsured squarely before the American public. The defeat of the Clinton health reform proposals meant that the problem remains in front of us, with no clear solution in sight. As shown in Figure 10.1, the percentage of uninsured Americans has grown nearly continuously since the Wofford and Clinton elections.

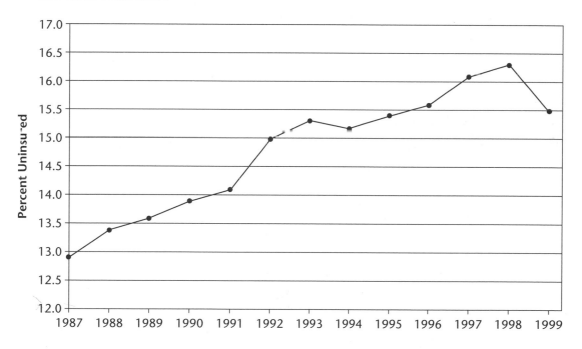

Figure 10.1 Percentage of U.S. Population Without Health Insurance, 1987–1999

When Harris Wofford campaigned in 1991 on the issue of national health insurance there were 35.4 million uninsured Americans. When the

Clinton health reform proposals were defeated in 1994 there were 39.7 million uninsured Americans. By 1998 this number had grown to 44.3 million people without insurance. Finally in 1999, after years of economic expansion and strikingly low rates of unemployment, the number of uninsured Americans dipped to 42.6 million, or 15.5% of the population. In order to understand why the number of people without health insurance grew continuously even in the face of one of the longest and strongest periods of economic growth in our country's history, it is necessary to understand who the uninsured are.

In looking at what type of people are uninsured, we will look only at those people in this country who were without health insurance for the entire year. In addition to the 44.3 million people who fell into this category in 1999, millions of others were without insurance for some period during the year, but not the entire year. Many people change jobs and are without coverage in the interim. Many college students go without health insurance coverage for short periods between graduation and beginning employment. People who are self-employed may cancel their coverage for a period of time and enroll with a new insurance carrier. These, however, are not the people we are talking about when we discuss the uninsured. The data below apply only to those who are without health insurance for the full year.

Figure 10.2 The Uninsured by Household Income, 1999
Source: U.S. Census Bureau

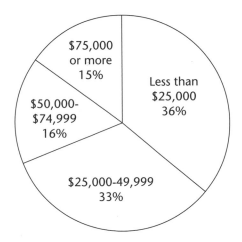

Figure 10.2 shows the breakdown of the population of uninsured Americans in 1999 by household income. The first thing to note is that only 36% of the uninsured come from low-income families (families with income less than $25,000). Nearly half of the uninsured are from families with household income between $25,000 and $75,000 per year.

Concept 10.2

The problem of the uninsured is not principally a problem affecting low-income families. Nearly two-thirds of uninsured Americans are in families with annual household income above $25,000.

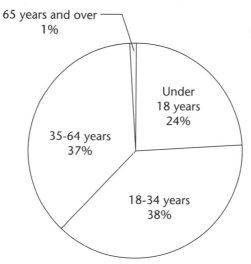

65 years and over
1%

35-64 years
37%

Under
18 years
24%

18-34 years
38%

Figure 10.3 The Uninsured by Age, 1999

Figure 10.3 looks at the uninsured by age. As would be expected, only 1% of the uninsured are elderly. Medicare has been very effective in maintaining nearly universal coverage for elderly Americans. Thirty-eight percent of the uninsured are young adults between 18 and 34. Nearly one in four of the uninsured is a child. This high rate of uninsured children persists despite expansions in Medicaid eligibility for children and creation of the CHIP program, an entirely new national program to offer health insurance to children. CHIP and its problems are discussed below.

Concept 10.3

The uninsured are made up mostly of young Americans. Twenty-four percent are children. Thirty-eight percent are young adults.

By looking at Figure 10.4 it is apparent that the uninsured are not distributed equally among the principal ethnic groups in the United States. In

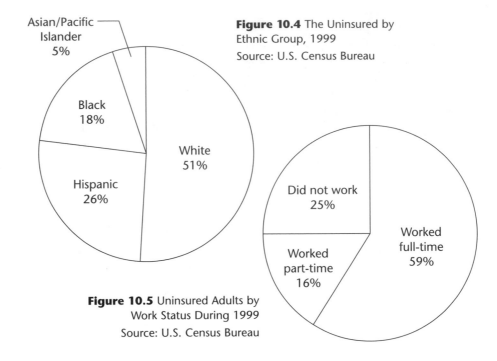

Figure 10.4 The Uninsured by Ethnic Group, 1999
Source: U.S. Census Bureau

Figure 10.5 Uninsured Adults by Work Status During 1999
Source: U.S. Census Bureau

Concept 10.4

Minority ethnic groups are overrepresented among the uninsured. This is especially true for Hispanics.

1999 72% of the U.S. population was white, but only 51% of the uninsured were white. The overall population was 12% black, but the uninsured were 18% black. The population was 12% Hispanic, but the uninsured were 26% Hispanic. Asian/Pacific Islanders made up 4% of the population and 5% of the uninsured. All major minority ethnic groups are overrepresented among the uninsured. The percentage of Hispanics among the uninsured is more than twice the percentage of Hispanics in the general population.

As shown in Figure 10.5, the problem of the uninsured is principally a problem of working families. During 1999 only 25% of uninsured adults did not work. Fifty-nine percent of the uninsured worked full-time during the year, with the remaining 16% working part-time.

From the above data, it is possible to draw the following conclusions. Those Americans who are uninsured are

- Principally young (52% under 35 years of age)

- Principally from minority ethnic groups (26% Hispanic and 18% black)
- Principally from middle-income, working families (59% of adults work full-time, 64% of families have incomes above $25,000 per year)

The problem of the uninsured is not primarily a problem of the poor and the unemployed. It is a problem of middle-class, working families. How is it that, with most people obtaining health insurance through their work, so many working Americans remain without coverage? To answer this question, we will look in detail at the employment characteristics of the uninsured.

The Source of the Uninsured: Low-Wage Workers and Small Employers

Not all workers have equal access to health insurance through their work. In addition, not all workers take advantage of the availability of health insurance at their work. The likelihood a worker will have coverage available and the likelihood the worker will accept coverage when offered seems to be closely associated with the worker's hourly wage. As Figure 10.6 shows, only 42.7% of workers who earn $7.00 or less are offered the chance to participate in employer-sponsored health insurance. For workers earning between $7.01 and $10.00 per hour the figure rises to 70%. Ninety-four percent of workers earning more than $15.00 per hour have health insurance offered to them through their work.

Even if an employer offers health insurance coverage to workers, not all workers accept this coverage. Typically the employer pays only part of the cost of coverage, with the employee responsible for paying the balance. It is possible to arrange to have the employee's share of the insurance premium exempt from income tax. However, for lower-wage workers the advantage of tax-exemption holds less benefit, since these workers typically pay taxes at a lower rate (if at all). In addition, the impact of the reduction in take-home pay resulting from enrolling in the employer's health insurance plan is greater for low-wage workers than for higher-wage workers. As a result, even when offered coverage through their work, low-wage workers choose to accept that coverage less often than their higher-wage counterparts. Of those earning $7.00 per hour or less who are offered health insurance, only 63% accept the offer and enroll in the employer's health plan. The comparable number for higher-wage workers is 82–86%.

The rate of health insurance coverage depends not only on the wage of the employee but also on the size of the firm in which the worker is employed. As Figure 10.7 shows, fewer than one-third of workers

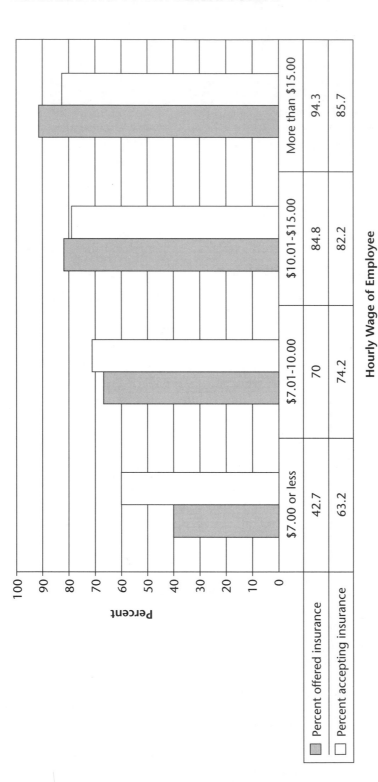

Figure 10.6 Availability and Acceptance of Employer-Sponsored Health Insurance for Workers at Different Income Levels, 1996

Source: Cooper and Schone, 1997

Concept 10.5

Low-wage workers are offered employer-sponsored health insurance less often and accept enrollment less often than higher-wage workers. As a result of the combination of these two forces, the rate of health insurance coverage is substantially lower among low-wage workers than higher-wage workers, even though many employers make coverage available.

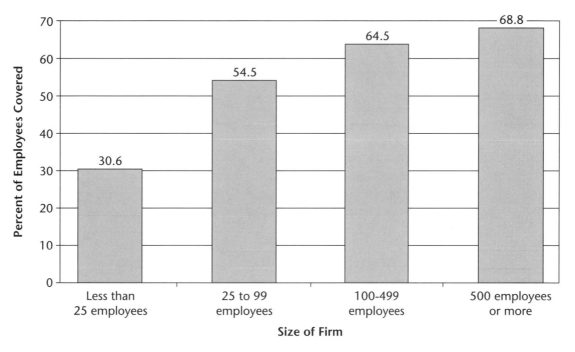

Figure 10.7 Percentage of Employees Covered by Employer-Sponsored Health Insurance, by Size of Firm, 1999
Source: U.S. Census Bureau

employed in firms with fewer than 25 employees are covered by employer-sponsored health insurance. Of employees in midsize firms, between 54% and 65% are covered. Nearly 70% of workers in firms with 500 employees or more are covered by the employer's plan.

There may well be substantial overlap between the effect of hourly wage and the effect of the size of the firm on the likelihood of coverage. Many small firms such as restaurants and independent retail stores rely on lower-wage workers to maintain their business. The cost of providing health insurance to these workers can be prohibitive. When Congress dis-

> ### Concept 10.6
>
> Workers in small firms (fewer than 25 employees) are less than half as likely as workers in large firms (500 employees or more) to be covered by employer-sponsored health insurance.

cussed requiring all employers to provide health insurance to their workers as part of the debate over the Clinton health reform proposals, small businesses spoke with a clear voice to say that such a mandate would be a severe hardship for them.

Our system of employer-based health insurance has evolved over several decades since the federal government made the two policy decisions described above. However, these decisions were intended to address specific issues of wage stabilization and taxation, and not to create national health policy. The system we have now was neither consciously designed nor explicitly adopted. It simply developed as a result of market forces and the unintended consequences of federal tax and wage policies. The system works well for most Americans. However, it has failed a growing segment of our population and has contributed substantially to the national policy dilemma of finding a way to extend coverage to the uninsured.

Two Programs to Reduce the Number of Uninsured

In recent years, two policies adopted on a limited basis have attempted to reduce the problem of the uninsured. The relative success of these programs offers valuable lessons about directions that future policies intended to reduce the number of uninsured might take. We examine each of these policies below.

Expanding Health Insurance Coverage in Hawaii: the Employer Mandate

For the years 1997–1999, only 9.5% of the population of the state of Hawaii was without health insurance coverage. Of all 50 states only Minnesota and Rhode Island had fewer uninsured. During this same period California had 21.3% of its population uninsured and Texas had 24.1% (U.S. Census Bureau 2000). Much of the credit for Hawaii's high rate of health insurance coverage for its population rests with the Prepaid Health Care Act (PPHCA), the country's only statewide employer-mandate system of health insurance.

In the 1970s the number of uninsured in Hawaii was typical of the rest of the United States: 12% of the population was without hospital insurance and 17% without insurance for physician care (Lewin and Sybinsky 1993). Seeing the rising cost of health care as a threat to the local population and the local economy, the Hawaii state legislature enacted PPHCA in 1974. Virtually all employers were required to provide health insurance for employees working at least half time. The cost of the insurance was to be paid by a payroll tax on employees (not to exceed 1.5% of wages), with the balance paid by the employer. With these funds the employer would purchase a basic health insurance policy, covering at least a specified list of services, from one of the private health insurance providers in the state. The mandated coverage would be for the employee only, but employers and employees would have the option of covering other family members. (Most employers have extended coverage to family members.)

The law was very successful, with between 4% and 5% of the population remaining without insurance by the mid-1980s. A serious economic downturn in Hawaii following the Asian currency crisis of the early 1990s led to higher rates of unemployment in the state. For example, the unemployment rate in Hawaii was 2.6% in January 1991 and rose to 6.4% in January 1997. In the same period the overall U.S. unemployment rate fell from 6.4% to 5.3% (data from the U.S. Bureau of Labor Statistics). As a result the number of uninsured in Hawaii climbed to over 9%. Even with this rise in unemployment relative to the rest of the country, Hawaii has one of the lowest uninsured rates of all 50 states. Those who remain without health insurance in Hawaii are part-time workers, the unemployed, and dependents of low-income workers.

It should be noted that the federal Employee Retirement Income Security Act (often referred to simply as ERISA) was enacted by Congress shortly after Hawaii created PPHCA. ERISA prohibits any other state from enacting an employer mandate. Thus Hawaii remains the only state with an employer mandate for health insurance.

Whenever an employer mandate to provide health insurance to workers is proposed, whether at the national or state level, the business community raises serious objections. The principal concern is that such a mandate would place an unreasonable burden on small businesses. Specifically, adding the cost of health insurance to the other costs of doing business might drive some firms out of business and lead others to scale back the number of people they are willing to employ. The result is predicted to be higher unemployment and reduced business activity. Similar predictions were made when PPHCA was first proposed in 1974.

These predictions did not prove to be accurate. A study by the federal government showed that PPHCA did not adversely affect businesses in

Hawaii (Lewin and Sybinsky 1993). More than 90% of businesses in Hawaii employ fewer than 50 people. In a state with one of the highest proportion of small businesses in the country, the creation of an employer mandate for the provision of health insurance did not appreciably harm small business owners or employees.

One aspect of the PPHCA that was particularly important, and which holds particular significance for consideration of the general policy issue of the employer mandate, was the experience with the Premium Supplementation Fund. Part of PPHCA is that employers with eight employees or fewer who are not able to afford the added costs of health insurance for workers are eligible to apply for state assistance in paying these premiums. In the first 17 years of the program only $85,000 was expended from this fund. Even the very smallest businesses in Hawaii seem to be able to comply with the employer mandate without undue hardship.

Concept 10.7

Requiring all employers to provide health insurance to their regular employees and their families has been demonstrated to reduce the number of uninsured substantially without imposing undue hardship on small businesses.

The experience of Hawaii with an employer mandate for health insurance suggests that this method of extending health insurance to all workers and their families can succeed. As a result of the federal government's prohibition on employer mandates elsewhere, the Hawaii experiment has not been duplicated elsewhere in the country. Nonetheless the concept of the employer mandate may hold substantial promise for addressing the problem of the uninsured.

CHIPing Away at the Number of Uninsured Children

As part of the national debate that arose following the victory of Harris Wofford in 1991 and the Clinton health reform proposals of 1993–1994, the number of uninsured children became a major national concern. Few had been aware that nearly 10 million children were without health insurance and as a result without access to basic medical care. A national consensus developed around this issue. Republicans and Democrats alike felt that, even if we as a country could find no solution to the general problem of the uninsured, we could at least find a way to extend basic coverage to children. Children, after all, are the least expensive age group to insure and can benefit the most from basic services such as immunizations and preventive care.

In 1997 a bipartisan coalition developed in Congress around this issue. In August 1997 Congress enacted the State Children's Health Insurance Program (P.L. 105-33), often referred to simply as CHIP, as Title XXI of the Social Security Act. Under CHIP a federal/state partnership was established with the goal of significantly reducing the number of uninsured children. The target population was uninsured children in families that were not previously eligible for Medicaid and that earned less than 200% of the federal poverty level.

Each state was given a financial incentive to create a new, statewide program for extending health insurance coverage to uninsured children. The states were given the option of three ways in which to do this. States could:

1. Expand the existing Medicaid program to include more children
2. Establish a program separate and distinct from Medicaid to extend coverage to those children not eligible for Medicaid
3. Use a combination of both Medicaid expansion and new program creation

CHIP appropriated between $3 billion and $5 billion per year for 10 years, with the explicit goal of cutting the number of uninsured children in half nationwide. States would design a program and apply to the federal government to have the majority of the costs of the program paid out of federal funds. The first CHIP funds became available to the states on October 1, 1997. Once allocated funds, a state had three years in which to spend the funds to provide health insurance for eligible children. After the three-year period, any funds not used for this purpose had to be returned to the federal government.

States responded enthusiastically to CHIP. Of the 56 states and territories eligible to participate, 51 had established plans by April 1999. The four states with largest number of uninsured children—California, Florida, New York, and Texas—were allocated nearly half of the available funding. States were almost evenly divided between those who used expansion of Medicaid on one hand and those who created a new program, either stand-alone or in combination with Medicaid, on the other.

The first two years of CHIP showed considerable success in meeting its stated goal of cutting the number of uninsured children in half. In December 1998, a year after the program was enacted, 833,303 children were covered under CHIP. By December 1999, 2 million previously uninsured children had obtained coverage through CHIP (data from HCFA).

However CHIP began to run into trouble in a number of states. Reports from state governments as well as children's advocacy agencies began to suggest that the enrollment of eligible children was lagging far behind projections in a number of areas. Some states were reluctant to invest state funds in the program, often leading to delays of up to a year in the opening of enrollment. Other states established application procedures that were so complex, many eligible families simply failed to apply. Other states failed to establish adequate outreach programs and were simply unable to find the eligible children they had hoped to enroll.

The three-year period in which states were required to spend their initial allocation of funds ended on September 30, 2000. Remaining funds that had not been spent by the states to provide coverage to children had to be returned to the federal government. Nearly half of the previously allocated money—$1.9 billion out of $4.2 billion—remained unspent by the states on September 30 (*New York Times,* September 2000). California had to return $590 million, or 69% of its original allocation. Texas had to return $446 million. New Mexico, with 30,000 uninsured children, could only enroll 1000 of these in its CHIP program and had to return 92% of its original allotment. Only 10 states were able to spend the full amount given to them by the federal government to enroll uninsured children in CHIP. Of these, New York was perhaps the most successful, with 550,000 new children enrolled, one-fourth of the national total.

Unfortunately New York's success in enrolling children was soon cast in another light. Shortly after the federal government reported the failure of the CHIP program overall to meet its enrollment goals but the success of New York program, newspapers reported that as many as half of the children enrolled in New York may not have actually been eligible for CHIP (*New York Times,* September 24, 2000). Federal law requires that uninsured children who are eligible for Medicaid must be enrolled by states in their existing Medicaid program and not in CHIP. The states pay a larger share of the cost of Medicaid, and Congress did not want them to shift Medicaid-eligible children into CHIP in order to gain a higher level of federal subsidy. It appears that this is precisely what New York did. As a result New York may also be required to return part of the funding it received.

The CHIP program was established by a bipartisan coalition in Congress to try to cut the number of uninsured children in half. It relied on the states

Concept 10.8

As exemplified by the Children's Health Insurance Program (CHIP), national policies to extend coverage to the uninsured that rely on states to implement and carry out new insurance programs may have problems attaining program goals.

to establish and carry out the programs to meet this goal. The states responded with ambivalence—they wanted to take advantage of the federal subsidy to cover more children, but they shied away from a full commitment either to the program or to the goal.

FURTHER READING

The history of the development of health insurance in America is described in detail in Paul Starr's book, *The Social Transformation of American Medicine* (Basic Books: New York, 1982). Information included here draws heavily on Book 2, Chapter 2 from that book. Students interested in learning more about the economic, political, and historical forces that shaped health care in America during the twentieth century are encouraged to read this Pulitzer Prize–winning work.

ON-LINE DATA SOURCES

Extensive information about the uninsured is available from the U.S. Census Bureau at www.census.gov/. Census Bureau data cited in this chapter come principally from the report Health Insurance Coverage 1999 (P60-211), issued in September 2000 and available at www.census.gov/hhes/www/hlthin99.html.

The Kaiser Family Foundation publishes numerous reports and data about the uninsured through its Kaiser Commission on Medicaid and the Uninsured, available at www.kff.org.

The U.S. Health Care Financing Administration has information about the CHIP program available at www.hcfa.gov/init/children.htm.

Unemployment data cited in this chapter are available from the U.S. Bureau of Labor Statistics at http://stats.bls.gov.

REFERENCES

Ayanian JZ, Weissman JS, Schneider EC, at al. Unmet Health Needs of Uninsured Adults in the United States. *JAMA* 2000; 284:2061–69.

Cooper PE, Schone BS. More Offers, Fewer Takers for Employment-Based Health Insurance: 1987 and 1996. *Health Affairs* 1997; 16(6):142–48.

Lewin JC, Sybinsky PA. Hawaii's Employer Mandate and Its Contribution to Universal Access. *JAMA* 1993; (269):2538–43.

Pear R. 40 States Forfeit Health Care Funds for Poor Children. *New York Times* September 24, 2000. National edition Section A, p. 1.

Steinhauer J. States Prove Unpredictable in Aiding Uninsured Children. *New York Times* September 28, 2000. National edition Section A, p. 16.

Steinhauer J. Many Not Eligible in State Program to Insure Children. *New York Times* September 30, 2000. National edition Section A, p. 1.

CHAPTER 11

Factors Other Than Health Insurance That Impede Access to Care

Key Concepts

- For patients with health insurance coverage, the type of insurance may affect access to care, with potential adverse health consequences.

- When patients are responsible for paying for part of their care, they are less likely to use that care. Having a 25% coinsurance rate led to a 16% reduction in the overall cost of care. It also led to a decrease in necessary as well as unnecessary care.

- Among male patients who came to a VA hospital for treatment of a heart attack, blacks were significantly less likely than whites to receive aggressive care involving revascularization. Although the lower rate of revascularization did not affect long-term survival, it did result in a lower quality of life for black patients.

- For a variety of serious medical conditions, and in a variety of settings and geographic locations, black patients receive less aggressive and lower quality care than white patients with the same disease, even after taking into account the type of insurance the patient has.

- As a result of subtle, often unconscious bias, physicians may treat patients from certain minority ethnic groups differently than comparable white patients. Although this bias may not necessarily constitute racism in the classical sense, it nonetheless can result in lower quality care for black and other minority patients.

- The large organizational systems that are typical of managed care tend to be more complex, more impersonal, and to have problems with patient satisfaction with care.

- Factors external to the actual doctor-patient interaction can exert a strong influence on patients' perceptions of the quality of the care they receive.

- "Unfortunately, the track record of American health care, especially in recent times, does not support the belief that coverage is equivalent to access" (Friedman 1994).

A s discussed in Chapter 10, the growing number of Americans with no health insurance is a major national problem. It will be difficult to address the problem without significant changes in health policy at both the state and federal levels. It is important, however, to understand that even if we are able to move to a system of universal health insurance, simply having health insurance does not always ensure full access to care. As complex as the issue of universal health insurance is, the issue of universal access is even more complex.

A number of barriers to accessing high-quality care have little to do with whether or not a patient has health insurance. These barriers generally stem from forces within the organizational environment of the health care delivery system or within the broader social system itself. In this chapter we examine a number of these forces and how they create barriers to full health care access.

Type of Health Insurance Coverage and Access to Care for Urgent Problems

Certain types of urgent medical problems, once diagnosed, have a well-defined treatment. Acute appendicitis is one such problem. Although it is not always easy to diagnose appendicitis, once diagnosed the treatment is clear: appendectomy (the surgical removal of the appendix). In addition, it is well known that delays in the diagnosis and treatment of appendicitis will increase the chances of developing a potentially serious complication: rupture of the appendix.

A study reported in 1994 (Braveman et al. 1994) asked the following question: Will the type of insurance a patient has affect the chances of developing a ruptured appendix for those patients with acute appendicitis? Appendicitis was studied for two reasons: (1) It is an illness that is not apparently affected by social or lifestyle factors, and thus can be expected to occur with approximately equal frequency for different socioeconomic groups: (2) Once diagnosed, it is promptly treated in almost all cases, regardless of insurance status. Thus, the key variable in whether a patient will have his appendix out before it ruptures is how easily the patient is able to obtain access to care. The study looked at this question for four groups, three of which had health insurance coverage:

- Patients with traditional fee-for-service insurance
- Patients with insurance through an HMO
- Patients on Medicaid
- Patients with no health insurance

The study had two important findings:

- Patients with either Medicaid or no insurance had approximately a 50% greater risk of developing a ruptured appendix than patients with HMO coverage.
- Patients with fee-for-service insurance were at a 20% greater risk of developing a ruptured appendix than those with HMO coverage.

For patients with Medicaid, it appears that the barriers to obtaining care for acute appendicitis are similar to the barriers faced by patients with no insurance at all. Lacking a regular source of care, both populations frequently have to rely on the emergency room of large, often crowded hospitals to obtain care for urgent problems. In this case simply having insurance does little to ensure prompt access.

It is interesting, though, that the patients with traditional, fee-for-service insurance also faced an increased chance of developing a ruptured appendix when compared to HMO patients. Though the difference between fee-for-service and HMO patients was smaller than that between Medicaid patients and HMO patients, it was nonetheless substantial. Why would patients with full insurance have problems obtaining prompt diagnosis and treatment for acute appendicitis?

Although the study did not definitively answer this question, there are two possible explanations. One is that patients with fee-for-service insurance do not automatically have a physician available to them as part of their insurance. They still have to seek out a physician on their own. Patients with full insurance but no established physician can face delays in obtaining care and may end up finding care in the emergency room. By comparison, patients with HMO insurance receive a list of providers from which to choose, and are often required to select a primary care physician at the time of their enrollment. Having a previously identified provider can facilitate obtaining care in an urgent situation.

Another explanation is that fee-for-service insurance often involves deductibles and copayments that the patient must pay. These out-of-pocket expenses are typically higher for fee-for-service patients than for patients with HMO coverage, and as a result may lead to patients delaying necessary care.

Concept 11.1

For patients with health insurance coverage, the type of insurance may affect the accessibility of care, with potential adverse health consequences.

In the following sections we look more closely at the way out-of-pocket expenses for health care can affect access to care and the effect of Medicaid coverage on access to care.

The Effect of Out-of-Pocket Expenses on the Rate at Which Patients Access Care

The Rand Health Insurance Experiment looked closely at the question of how the amount a patient has to pay out of pocket to obtain care affects the frequency with which the patient seeks care. This study demonstrated an association between the amount a patient must pay and the frequency with which the patient actually will obtain care (Newhouse et al. 1981). The study looked at people who were randomly assigned to one of four different insurance plans, each with a different level of payment required from the patient:

1. Patient pays nothing out of pocket
2. Patient pays 25% of all charges
3. Patient pays 50% of all charges
4. Patient pays 95% of all charges.

The percentage of the cost that the patient must pay is called the "coinsurance rate." In plans 2–4 the patient had a yearly cap of $1000 in out-of-pocket expenditures. After that amount, all additional care was 100% covered. Table 11.1 shows the results of this study, comparing the frequency with which the patient visited the doctor and the overall cost of care for different coinsurance rates.

Table 11.1

Effect of Coinsurance on Use and Annual Cost of Services: Rand Health Insurance Study

Level of Insurance	Doctor's Office Visits per Year	Total Yearly Expenditures
Free care	5.4	$401
25% Coinsurance	4.4	$346
50% Coinsurance	3.2	$328
95% Coinsurance	3.7	$254

Source: Newhouse et al. 1981

It can be seen that the amount of coinsurance a patient faces affects both the frequency with which the patient visits the doctor and the overall cost of care (including both doctor care and hospital care) for that patient. Patients with free care visited the doctor 23% more often than those with 25% coinsurance and 69% more than patients with 50% coinsurance.

These findings raise the following question: Will coinsurance prevent patients from seeking needed care? The researchers looked at the types of outpatient visits and hospitalizations the different groups made, using a panel of experts to categorize the care received (or forgone) as necessary or unnecessary. They found that those with higher coinsurance had fewer visits and hospitalizations characterized as necessary as well as those characterized as unnecessary. From this study we can conclude the following about the effect of coinsurance on the use of care.

Concept 11.2

When patients are responsible for paying for part of their care, they are less likely to use that care. Having a 25% coinsurance rate led to a 14% reduction in the overall cost of care. It also led to a decrease in necessary as well as unnecessary care.

The Effect of Medicaid Coverage on Patients' Access to Care

As noted in Chapter 6, patients with Medicaid insurance may still have problems accessing care:

- Due to low reimbursement rates, only one-third of doctors have been willing to accept new Medicaid patients in their practice.

- In many communities so few doctors are willing to see Medicaid patients that the only regular source of care is the hospital emergency room.

The Braveman study cited earlier also showed that

- Medicaid patients have difficulty accessing care for acute appendicitis, leading to a rate of ruptured appendix that is 50% greater than for HMO patients.

A 1994 study took a detailed look at the experience Medicaid patients face in trying to obtain medical care for common problems (Medicaid Access Study Group 1994). Researchers called a wide variety of private doctors' offices, hospital-based clinics, and community clinics in several locales.

The caller posed as a Medicaid patient and asked to obtain care for a common, relatively minor type of complaint (low back pain, bladder infection, sore throat). They asked if they could be seen for this problem, and if so, how quickly. The researchers let a few weeks go by, and then they called back many of these same offices and clinics, this time posing as someone with full private insurance. They asked for an appointment for the same problem as the Medicaid caller. They recorded how many of the doctors or clinics were willing to see them, and how soon they could be seen. The results are shown in Table 11.2.

Table 11.2   Results of the Study of Medicaid Access to Care

Response to Medicaid recipients	
Able to make any appointment	44%
Appointment available within 2 days	35%
Appointment available after 5 PM	13%
Response to patient with private insurance	
Appointment available within 2 days	60%

Source: Medicaid Access Study Group 1994

Having Medicaid insurance does not guarantee access to care. The move to managed care for state Medicaid programs may ameliorate this problem somewhat. However, any state or national policy proposal that seeks to extend health insurance coverage to those currently uninsured by expanding the Medicaid program will have to cope with this problem of access.

Racial Barriers to Health Care Access

Throughout much of the twentieth century the United States maintained a health care system that, in many parts of the country, divided access to care along racial lines: the race of the patient as well as the race of the doctor. There were separate hospitals for black patients and white patients. Even those doctors and clinics that agreed to treat both groups of patients often maintained separate waiting rooms for black and white patients. Separate medical schools were created to train black doctors. With the official sanctioning of national and local medical societies, fully qualified black doctors were prevented from joining the medical staff of white hospitals.

In the 1960s, as part of the civil rights movement and landmark civil rights legislation, the federal government took action against this segregated system of care. Hospitals that maintained policies for segregated treatment and medical staff were ineligible to obtain federal payment through the Medicare and Medicaid programs. Over the period of a few years the segregated system of care was largely dismantled. Black patients and black doctors finally obtained access to previously all-white institutions.

The hope was that by desegregating the health care system our country could attain a level of care that, though still depending on a patient's ability to pay, otherwise treated all patients equally. Unfortunately the last several years have produced a continuing litany of evidence that we have not yet met this goal. One of the first studies that pointed to continuing racial barriers in access to care looked at the way in which patients receive care for heart attacks in the federal Veterans' Affairs (VA) health system.

The VA operates a series of hospitals throughout the United States. Many of these hospitals are affiliated with academic medical centers. Eligibility for care depends on a patient having served in the American armed forces and meeting certain income requirements. Once deemed eligible, any veteran may receive free hospital care.

A study looked closely at the experience of male patients, all eligible for VA care, who came to a VA hospital in the years 1988–1990 with a heart attack (Peterson et al. 1994). At that time it was common practice at most hospitals, including VA hospitals, to consider all patients with an acute heart attack for a procedure called cardiac revascularization. Since a heart attack is caused by a blocked artery in the heart, using a surgical procedure to reopen the blocked blood vessel can improve the patient's outcome. There are two principal types of revascularization procedures:

- Angioplasty, in which a thin balloon is inserted into the blocked vessel and the vessel is reopened by inflating the balloon
- Coronary artery bypass graft surgery (referred to as CABG), in which a section of blood vessel is taken from the patient's leg and surgically implanted into the blocked vessel in a way that bypasses the blockage

Before either procedure is done the patient undergoes cardiac catheterization, in which dye is injected directly into the arteries of the heart and X rays are taken, showing the exact location and size of the blockage. The VA study examined whether black patients and white patients, all coming to a VA hospital with a heart attack, receive different levels of treatment. After controlling for individual characteristics of the patients (age, other illness, etc.), the study came to the following conclusions:

- Blacks were 33% less likely than whites to undergo cardiac catheterization.
- Blacks were 42% less likely than whites to undergo angioplasty.

- Blacks were 54% less likely than whites to undergo CABG surgery.
- Blacks were 54% less likely than whites to undergo any type of revascularization procedure.

The study then went on to look at the likelihood a patient would survive his heart attack, examining whether the demonstrated differences in access to revascularization procedures were associated with differences in survival. It came to some very interesting conclusions:

- In the first 30 days after the heart attack, survival among black patients was significantly higher than among white patients.
- At one year and two years after the heart attack there was no difference in survival among whites and blacks.
- In terms of the quality of life for patients who did survive the heart attack, surviving black patients had more chest pain and a lower overall quality of life than white patients.

Concept 11.3

Among male patients who came to a VA hospital for treatment of a heart attack, blacks were significantly less likely than whites to receive aggressive care involving revascularization. Although the lower rate of revascularization did not affect long-term survival, it did result in a lower quality of life for black patients.

Since the VA heart study came out, a number of additional studies have reported racial differences in access to care, painting a disturbing picture. Among the findings are the following:

- Black patients with heart disease and other serious health problems receive less aggressive and lower quality care, even after taking into account the type of insurance the patient has (Kahn et al. 1994; Ayanian, Weissman et al. 1999).
- Black patients with early-stage lung cancer (a stage at which patients have a higher chance of cure if treated appropriately) are treated less aggressively, with lower rates of surgery than comparable white patients (Bach et al. 1999).
- Black patients with kidney failure who are receiving regular kidney dialysis (and thus are automatically eligible for Medicare insurance coverage) are referred less often than white patients for consideration of kidney transplantation (Ayanian, Cleary, et al. 1999).

- Despite a higher incidence among the black population of a form of bone marrow cancer called multiple myeloma, blacks with the disease receive bone marrow transplantation less often than whites, despite the evidence that this treatment substantially prolongs survival (Boyce 2000).

- Both black patients (Todd et al. 2000) and Hispanic patients (Todd et al. 1993) who receive emergency treatment for broken bones receive less pain medication while in the emergency room than white patients with similarly broken bones.

Concept 11.4

For a variety of serious medical conditions, and in a variety of settings and geographic locations, black patients receive less aggressive and lower quality care than white patients with the same disease, even after taking into account the type of insurance the patient has.

The question arises as to whether other ethnic minorities face the same disadvantages as blacks in obtaining full and equal access to care. Fewer studies have been done looking at Hispanics, Native Americans, Asians, and other ethnic groups, so we don't fully know the answer to this question. Future research will need to be done to understand whether racially based differences in access to care also exist for other ethnic groups.

Decades after the federally mandated integration of health care facilities in this country, the issue of racial bias in our medical care system persists. Why are black patients denied access to the same level of care as white patients? Might it be that physicians in this country are biased in the way they approach patients from differing ethnic groups?

The question of racial bias on the part of physicians raises important ethical issues, yet often triggers powerful emotional responses. This dilemma is not unique to medical care. Whether in housing, employment, education, or health care, the history of racial discrimination in the United States evokes memories of reprehensible behavior on the part of individuals and governments, often involving hatred and open hostility toward blacks and other minorities.

However, intentional, explicit racism of this type is probably not the most likely explanation of the widespread racial differences we continue to see in treatment and outcomes. Approaching racial bias as a single, uniform phenomenon inappropriately simplifies what is a complex, multifaceted set of psychological mechanisms. Racial bias can exist and exert its effects on many levels and in many ways, even in people who would honestly be horrified to have racist beliefs attributed to them. Hatred and overt bigotry represent only one type of bias, although this form of bias is what most people think of when the issue is discussed. We can identify other mechanisms that do not involve conscious racism but which nonetheless can lead to differences in the treatment of members of differing racial groups.

Before describing these forms of unintended bias, however, it is important to acknowledge that the concept of race and the grouping of people according to racial characteristics do not reflect genetic differences but rather social constructions. It is not possible to identify a set of genetic markers that reliably separate people into what we have come to understand as races (e.g., black, white). There is more genetic variability within "races" than between races. Nonetheless, people continue to act as though race were a valid means of categorizing people. See Anderson (2001) and Goodman (2000) for a more detailed discussion of these issues.

Statistical Bias

Statistical bias involves an individual making a seemingly rational decision based on data about differences in behavior among racial groups. The example of the inner-city taxi driver illustrates statistical bias. In deciding whether to pick up a potential customer, is it justifiable to consider the race of the customer? The incidence of robbery is higher among black taxi customers than among white customers. Can we blame the driver who passes up a black man hailing the cab and picks up a white man instead?

In choosing to pick up the white customer, the cab driver is assigning a stereotyped group characteristic to an individual perceived to be a member of that group. In this case the perceived group is all blacks living in the area where the driver works; the pertinent group characteristic is the probability the customer will attempt to rob the driver. The driver has no information pertaining specifically to the potential customer other than racial appearance. nonetheless an argument can be made that in the absence of other information, it is "rational" to assign the group characteristic to the individual.

A decision of this type, based on principles of rationality, can lead to unequal outcomes for racial groups. The unequal outcomes do not necessarily invalidate the decision. However, in some contexts, for certain public purposes, we can preclude the application of statistical inference based on racial groupings. In New York City, for example, cab drivers are enjoined from racial differentiation among customers based on the overriding public need to have transportation by cab equally available to all.

In the medical care setting, statistical bias can exist in many ways. For example, many physicians consider the potential for patient compliance in deciding whether to recommend certain types of procedures. Kidney specialists, for example, may believe that black patients are more likely than white patients to have difficulty in following the stringent medication schedule required to prevent rejection after a kidney transplant and may in response hesitate in referring those patients for transplantation. In attributing the likelihood of noncompliance to a patient based on racial grouping, the kidney specialist creates the same fundamental situation as the cab driver. The public value of treating people as individuals in matters as crucial as the availability of organ transplantation (or cardiac revascularization, or cancer treatment) overrides the validity of assigning clinical characteristics to individual patients based on group inference.

Unconscious Bias

There is considerable empirical evidence that even self-described color-blind individuals can manifest racially discriminatory attitudes of which they are unaware (Dovidio and Gaertner 1998, vanRyn and Burke 2000). Although these people openly endorse fair and equal treatment of all racial groups and disavow overt racism, they harbor some type of negative feelings or association toward blacks or other minorities. When interacting with someone of a different race, they may feel discomfort on an unconscious level. They may express this discomfort in subtle ways that can have the effect of disadvantaging minority groups. Despite their biased actions, people acting on this unconscious level are not racists, but rather are acting based on cultural preferences learned long ago. (See Calman 2000 for a description of how this type of bias affected one patient in particular.)

A study in the medical literature concludes that physicians, without necessarily being conscious of personal bias, react differently to patients, and recommend different levels of treatment, based on the race or sex of the patient (Schulman et al. 1999). The study's authors showed a large sample of practicing physicians a videotape of an interview with a patient with possible heart disease. The subject was asked to assess the potential severity of the patient's condition and the need for aggressive care. The patients on the tapes were actually actors reading a script. Based purely on this scripted information, the physicians who saw the tapes, in aggregate, recommended that black patients receive less aggressive care than whites, and women less than men.

A follow-up study also demonstrated that first- and second-year medical students adopt a more aggressive approach to a diagnosing a white male patient with heart disease than a black female patient, even though each was an actor reading the same script (Rathore et al. 2000). The unconscious bias that may lead to racially based differences in treatment appears to exist even before physicians receive their clinical training.

> ## Concept 11.5
>
> As a result of subtle, often unconscious bias, physicians may treat patients from certain minority ethnic groups differently than comparable white patients. Although this bias may not necessarily constitute racism in the classical sense, it nonetheless can result in lower quality care for black and other minority patients.

Living Conditions and Care

It is well recognized that certain types of economic and living conditions can affect the health of individuals and social groups. Can living conditions also affect the way in which patients access care? This question can be answered, at least in part, by considering two separate studies looking at poor children with asthma.

The first study looked at differences in the way black children and white children with asthma use health services (Lozano et al. 1995). The study considered only children who were covered by Medicaid. All children in the study lived in the same city, had the same insurance coverage, and had access to the same hospitals and clinics. It found that black children go to the doctor's office less frequently yet have higher use of the emergency room and the hospital. Something other than insurance leads to these black children with asthma being sicker than their white counterparts, and to their relying more on the emergency room for care than the doctor's office.

The second study was an ingenious one (Rosenstreich et al. 1997). The researchers thought that there might be something in the bedroom of poor children that could cause an allergic reaction in some children, triggering an asthma attack. They took a group of poor children with asthma and tested them for allergy to three typical components of house dust: cat dander, dust mites, and cockroach droppings. The researchers then went into the bedroom of each of the children in the study and vacuumed up all the dust they could find. They took the dust to the laboratory and analyzed it for these same three components.

The study found that those children who were both allergic to cockroaches and had cockroaches in their bedroom were significantly sicker with their asthma than other children. Neither children with bedroom cockroaches but no allergy to cockroaches nor children who were allergic to cockroaches but had no cockroaches in their bedroom had as much problem with their asthma as those children with both conditions. The combination of cat or dust mite allergy and cat dander or dust mites in the bedroom did not seem to affect children nearly as much.

It appears that cockroaches in the home may have a lot to do with the pattern asthma takes in poor children. Although there were no data about the presence or absence of cockroaches in the bedroom of the children in the first study, one has to wonder whether the differences in the pattern of illness and medical care for poor black and white children with asthma may have to do, at least in part, with differences in the living conditions of black and white families.

Other Factors That May Affect Access to Care

Location

Many patients in rural areas simply are not as close to health care facilities, an access problem that is unaffected by insurance. The growing difficulty for rural hospitals to survive financially may lead to increased differences in access to care for urban and rural populations. Similarly, the relative scarcity of health care services and facilities in inner-city areas and other low-income neighborhoods makes access difficult even for those with insurance. Problems with transportation, arranging child care, and taking take time off work to seek care may all contribute to geographic differences in access to care.

Culture

Language frequently presents a barrier to obtaining care. Patients who do not have facility in speaking English may find it difficult to find a source of care. In addition, cultural belief systems about the nature of illness may delay obtaining care. Culturally based concerns about personal privacy and the embarrassment of physical examination by a stranger (often of a different sex) all can delay care.

Diagnosis

Many physicians and other health care providers are resistant to treating patients with AIDS. Similarly, many providers may feel very uncomfortable treating people with chronic mental illness for their physical problems. Drug and alcohol abusers have many very real physical problems, yet many providers do not want to treat these patients.

The Increasing Organizational Complexity of Health Care as a Barrier to Care

Our system of health care has moved from one based on fee-for-service care provided largely by independent doctors in relatively small offices and groups to one in which care is provided on a capitation basis by systems of care involving large groups of physicians. In many cases physicians have shifted from being independent health care professionals to employees of large systems of care. Unfortunately, these changes have contributed to a growing sense of breakdown in the relationship between the physician and the patient. Nowhere is this more true that at the primary care level.

Maintaining high quality in primary care delivery depends largely on maintaining a strong relationship between the doctor and the patient. From a variety of research it has been possible to identify factors that create a satisfying doctor/patient relationship from the perspective of the patient.

- *Humanistic behavior by physicians.* Patients need to have a sense that the doctor cares about them as a person and will take the time to listen to and understand their concerns.

- *Caring interpersonal interaction with other employees.* Patients need to be treated in a sensitive and courteous manner by the other employees who work with the doctor.

- *Continuity of care.* Patients need to develop an ongoing relationship with a physician they can count on seeing over a period of time.

- *Accessibility of care.* Patients need to be able to arrange to see their physician in a timely manner when the need arises, and to be able to get through to the doctor's office easily by phone.

- *Physician satisfaction with work conditions.* In order to be fully satisfied with their relationship with their physician, patients need to have a sense that their physician is also satisfied in the work he or she does. There appears to be a strong correlation between patient satisfaction with the quality of their relationship with their physician and physician satisfaction with work conditions.

When patients are asked what constitutes high quality in primary care, they usually describe the factors listed above. The technical competence of the physician seems to be less important than the humanistic competence, at least at the level of primary care. Thus patient satisfaction has emerged as a principal measure of primary care quality. Although health care regulators and health care managers who measure quality may look at the technical competence of the physician and the extent to which the physician follows standard procedures, patients tend to look more at the strength of their personal relationship with their doctor.

Unfortunately, throughout the history of HMOs and other types of managed care delivery systems, reductions in the cost of care have often been at the expense of reductions in the quality of primary care as measured by patient satisfaction. Recall from Chapter 4 that in both the Rand Health Insurance Experiment (Table 4.2) and the Medical Outcomes Study

(Table 4.3), HMOs score significantly lower than traditional fee-for-service systems on issues of the interpersonal nature of care, access to care, and continuity of care. As managed care delivery systems have become the rule rather than the exception, problems in patient satisfaction similar to those identified in these research studies have become more widespread. Looking at the changes in American health care that have accompanied the managed care revolution, one group of authors concluded, "Our patients want high quality service and do not believe they receive it" (Kenagy et al. 1999).

Why would a change in the way health care is organized and financed lead to a decrease in the quality of the relationship between the patient and the physician? In order to answer this question we need to understand some general principles of organizations theory (Barr 1995). Two characteristics of managed care are especially pertinent in this regard: the increasing size of medical practice groups that typically comes with a shift to managed care and the strengthening of management controls over certain aspects of medical practice.

In general, as an organization such as a medical practice group increases in size it tends to become more complex internally. This complexity involves increasing task specialization, with individual workers performing a more narrow range of duties. For example, in a smaller medical practice one person may answer the phones, greet patients, and make appointments, but in a larger group each task is done by a separate person. Task specialization often leads to increasingly complex paths of communication and to a more complex process for the customer (in this case the patient) to interact with the organization.

Added to the increased organizational complexity associated with increased organizational size is the effect on the medical care process of strengthened management systems. The capitation method of payment for health care requires that someone manage the provision of care to stay within the established budget. No individual practitioner has a sufficiently broad perspective to keep track of how available resources are being spent and how the demand for care is being met. Managed care as it is currently constructed requires a set of managers and management tools that are sufficiently removed from the care process to maintain direction and control of organizational activities.

Such a management structure creates potential conflict when the purpose of the organization is to provide a human service such as health care. As with other human services, health care, particularly at the primary care level, is based on high-quality interaction between the provider and the patient. Although cognizant of the need for strong provider-patient interaction, managers of a human service organization nonetheless tend to emphasize efficiency in the work of the organization. Efficiency in this context is often measured in units of production per unit of time (e.g., patients seen per hour). It is difficult to provide high-quality human service while under pressure to be efficient.

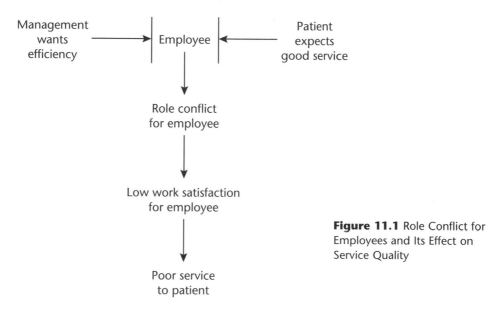

Figure 11.1 Role Conflict for Employees and Its Effect on Service Quality

Figure 11.1 illustrates the conflict between the desire to provide good service and the pressure to work efficiently that physicians in large managed care settings often encounter. This type of role conflict, however, often extends beyond the physician to encompass all types of employees who interact directly with patients. In general these workers want to be able to provide good service to patients, having chosen a service occupation over other alternatives. They, too, often face pressure to work more quickly and efficiently, based on management's need to maintain the efficiency of overall organizational processes. This situation has the potential to lead to what is described as role conflict: the conflict faced by a worker caught between the patient's desire for good service and management's emphasis on efficient work. Role conflict often leads to decreased worker satisfaction and a tendency to become less sensitive to the needs of patients.

The sum of these effects associated with the larger organizations increasingly typical of managed care is the potential for a less satisfactory experience for patients. In the managed care setting, patients often encounter systems that tend to be more complex and impersonal than the smaller types of medical groups that predominated under the traditional fee-for-service system. The problems in patient satisfaction associated with large managed care systems such as those studied in the Rand Health Insurance Experiment and the Medical Outcomes Study may have been caused by these types of characteristics.

> ## Concept 11.6
>
> The large organizational systems that are typical of managed care tend to be more complex, more impersonal, and to have problems with patient satisfaction with care.

In my own research I have looked at the extent to which factors within the organizational environment of a large primary care delivery system can affect patients' perceptions of the quality of their direct interaction with the physician (Barr et al. 2000). Using a survey questionnaire that has come to be widely used in medical practice (American Medical Group Association 2001), we asked a series of 291 patients who visited a primary care doctor the following questions about their visit.

In terms of your satisfaction, how would you rate each of the following?
- *The time spent with the doctor you saw*
- *Explanation of what was done for you*
- *The technical skills of the doctor you saw*
- *The personal manner of the doctor you saw*

Each question was answered on a 5-point scale, ranging from excellent to poor. We also asked patients to rate the quality of their interaction with the nurses and receptionists they encountered during their visit, using the same 5-point scale. When we analyzed the data, we found that 20% of the variation in the way patients rated their satisfaction with their direct interaction with the physician could be explained by two main factors:

- How courteously they were treated by the nurses and receptionists, and
- How long they had to wait at the doctor's office to see the doctor.

> ## Concept 11.7
>
> Factors external to the actual doctor-patient interaction can exert a strong influence on patients' perceptions on the quality of the care they receive.

This chapter has identified a variety of factors that can impede access to medical care. These factors have little to do with whether a patient does or does not have health insurance. Issues as divergent as geographic location, cultural norms, racial bias, and organizational complexity can get in the way of patients having full access to medical care. Since access to care is one of the key components of quality of care, any discussion of new policies for the organization, financing, and delivery of care should include this important principle.

Concept 11.8

"Unfortunately, the track record of American health care, especially in recent times, does not support the belief that coverage is equivalent to access" (Friedman 1994).

REFERENCES

American Medical Group Association. Visit-Specific Patient Satisfaction Survey. http://www.amga.org/AMGA2000/QMR/PSAT/survey_psat.htm Accessed 7/6/01.

Anderson, Elizabeth. Race, Gender, and Affirmative Action. University of Michigan. http://www-personal.umich.edu/~eandersn/biblio.htm Accessed 7/6/01.

Ayanian JZ, Weissman JS, Chasen-Taber S, Epstein AM. Quality of Care by Race and Gender for Congestive Heart Failure. *Medical Care* 1999; 37:1260–69.

Ayanian JZ, Cleary PD, Weissman JS, Epstein AM. The effect of patients' preferences on racial differences in access to renal transplantation. *New England Journal of Medicine* 1999; 341:1661-69.

Bach PB, Cramer LD, Warren JL, Begg CB. Racial Differences in the Treatment of Early-Stage Lung Cancer. *New England Journal of Medicine* 1999; 341:1198–1205

Barr DA. The Effect of Organizational Structure on Primary Care Outcomes Under Managed Care. *Annals of Internal Medicine* 1995; 122:353–59.

Barr DA, Vergun P, Barley SA. Problems in Using Patient Satisfaction Data to Assess the Quality of Care of Primary Care Physicians. *Journal of Clinical Outcomes Management* 2000; 7(9):1–6.

Boyce EA. Access to Bone Marrow Transplants for Multiple Myeloma Patients: The Role of Race. Thesis submitted for senior honors, Program in Human Biology, Stanford University, May 16, 2000.

Braveman P, Schaafrm, Egerter S, et al. Insurance Related Differences in the Risk of Ruptured Appendix. *New England Journal of Medicine* 1994; 331: 444–449.

Calman NS. Out of the Shadow. *Health Affairs* 2000; 19(1):170–74.

Dovidio J, Gaertner S. On the Nature of Contemporary Prejudice: The Causes, Consequences, and Challenges of Aversive Racism. In Eberhardt J, Fiske S, eds. *Confronting Racism: The Problem and the Response*. Thousand Oaks, Calif.: Sage Publications, 1998.

Friedman E. Money Isn't Everything: Nonfinancial Barriers to Access. *JAMA* 1994; 271:1535–38.

Goodman AH. Why Genes Don't Count (for Racial Differences in Health). *American Journal of Public Health* 2000; 90:1699–1702.

Kahn KL, Pearson ML, Harrison ER, et al. Health care for black and poor hospitalized Medicare patients. *JAMA* 1994; 271:1169–74.

Kenagy JW, Berwick DM, Shore MF. Service Quality in Health Care. *JAMA* 1999; 281:661–65.

Lozano P, Connell FA, Koepsell TD. Use of Health Services by African-American Children with Asthma on Medicaid. *JAMA* 1995; 274:469–73.

Medicaid Access Study Group. Access of Medicaid Recipients to Outpatient Care. *New England Journal of Medicine* 1994; 330:1426–30.

Newhouse JP, Manning WG, Morris CN, et al. Some Interim Results from a Controlled Trial of Cost Sharing in Health Insurance. *New England Journal of Medicine* 1981; 305:1501–7.

Peterson ED, Wright SM, Daley J, Thibault GE. Racial variation in cardiac procedure use and survival following acute myocardial infarction in the Department of Veterans Affairs. *JAMA* 1994; 271:1175–80.

Rathore SS, Lenert LA, Weinfurt KP, et al. The Effect of Patient Sex and Race on Medical Students' Ratings of Quality of Life. *American Journal of Medicine* 2000; 108:561–66.

Rosenstreich DL, Eggleston P, Kattan M, et al. The role of cockroach allergy and exposure to cockroach allergen in causing morbidity among inner-city children with asthma. *New England Journal of Medicine* 1997; 336:1356–63.

Schulman KA, Berlin JA, Harless W, et al. The effect of race and sex on physicians' recommendations for cardiac catheterization. *New England Journal of Medicine* 1999; 340:618–26.

Todd KH, Samaroo N, Hoffman JR. Ethnicity as a Risk Factor for Inadequate Emergency Department Analgesia. *JAMA* 1993; 269: 1537–39.

Todd KH, Deaton C, D'Adamo AP, Goe L. Ethnicity and Analgesic Practice. *Annals of Emergency Medicine* 2000; 35:11–16.

vanRyn M, Burke J. The effect of patient race and socio-economic status on physicians' perceptions of patients. *Social Science and Medicine* 2000; 50: 813–28.

CHAPTER 12

Where Do We Go From Here?

Key Concepts

- Rationing involves the prioritized allocation of scarce resources.
- The Oregon Health Plan did not create rationing where none previously existed. It instead shifted state policy from rationing health care based on income to rationing care based on need.
- The health care system in the United States involves rationing health care according to income. In contrast to the Oregon Health Plan, this rationing is implicit, with no explicit decision to ration care ever having been agreed to.
- You can treat some of the people all of the time, or you can treat all of the people some of the time, but you can't treat all of the people all of the time (Barr's law).

1. The cost of health care is higher in the United States than anywhere else in the world. After a period of relative stability these costs appear to be on the rise again.

2. The American public has largely come to expect the highest quality care available, regardless of the cost. Attempts to hold down the cost of care by constraining the availability of care have been met with resistance on many fronts.

3. The United States is the only industrialized country in the world that does not guarantee access to health care for all its citizens. An increasing segment of the American population lives without even basic health insurance, with negative consequences for access to care and quality of care.

These three principles, each addressed earlier in this book, largely define the problem facing policy makers, health care managers, health care providers, and patients alike. Each issue is pressing in its own right. Each deserves our attention. The conundrum of American health care is that all three exist simultaneously, and that attempting to remedy one will inevitably affect the others.

The problem of American health care can be represented by an equilateral triangle. As illustrated in Figure 12.1, each point of the triangle represents one of these fundamental policy issues: cost, quality, or access.

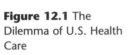

Figure 12.1 The Dilemma of U.S. Health Care

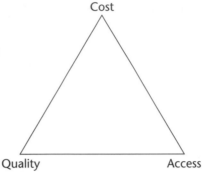

Imagine that the triangle is made out of cardboard and that it is situated horizontally. It is possible to find a single point of balance for this cardboard triangle. Once you find this balance point it is possible to balance the triangle on your finger. So long as you leave the triangle alone it will remain in balance. Now try to move one of the points of the triangle either up or down. Moving any one point in this manner will inevitably cause the other points to move.

The same is true for our health care system. As soon as we try to address one of the fundamental problems facing the system we find that our proposed solution will affect the other parts of the system, often adversely. Consider the following.

- If we try to control the cost of care, we will either reduce the quality of the care by making fewer services available or further decrease access to care by providing health insurance coverage to fewer people.

- If we try to improve access by expanding insurance coverage to those who are currently uninsured we will further increase the overall cost of care. Attempts to improve access while also attempting to hold down cost will impair quality.

- Attempts to improve the quality of care by introducing new treatments, technologies, or medications will add to the cost of the health care system, with the risk of driving more people into the ranks of the uninsured.

For decades the American health care system was like the triangle, perched on its balance point, albeit somewhat unsteadily. Although serious problems remained in our system, we had achieved a rough equilibrium between the competing needs of cost, quality, and access. The extension of health insurance to the elderly and the poor through the federal Medicare and Medicaid programs of the 1960s coincided with the beginnings of the explosion in medical technology. Attempts to hold down the cost of care through the expansion of HMOs led to the growing perception that quality was being impaired in ways that were unacceptable. Each point of our triangle had the forces of social and political change tugging at it. As a result our health care system was thrown out of balance and today continues to wobble precariously.

How are we to gain control of our health care system in a way that adequately addresses and balances competing problems and needs? This is the dilemma of American health care.

Victor Fuchs, one of the founders of the discipline of health economics, described our dilemma accurately and succinctly: "No pain—no gain" (Fuchs 1993). He points out that the issue of health care costs can be seen as simple arithmetic, represented by the equation illustrated in Figure 12.2.

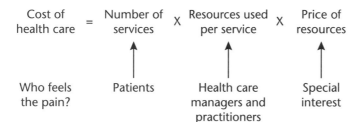

Figure 12.2 Health Care Costs Too Much—So How Can We Reduce Costs?

Source: Based on Fuchs 1993

In order to calculate overall health care costs, one simply has to multiply the following three numbers.

1. *The number of services provided to patients.* This includes the number of office visits, the number of hospitalizations, the number of operations, the number of tests, and the number of medications.

2. *The number of resources used in producing each service.* Here is where the issue of technology enters in so clearly. Does the doctor's office include all types of new, high-tech apparatus? Does the hospital include all the latest monitoring and diagnostic equipment? Will an operation incorporate laser scalpels and fiber-optics? Will we rely on newer, high-tech and usually high-priced medications over less expensive standbys?

3. *The price of the various resources used in providing services.* How much will we pay doctors for their care? How much will we pay hospitals? Will we allow the producers of medical equipment and pharmaceutical products to charge whatever the market will bear?

It is a simple fact of arithmetic that in order to reduce the cost of health care we will have to reduce at least one of the numbers appearing on the right side of the equation. The problem is, whenever we reduce one of these numbers, someone feels pain. When someone feels pain, they generally complain.

- If we try to reduce the number of services provided to patients, patients will perceive the reduction as a decrease in quality. Recent history has shown that, in response to constraints on the availability of services inherent in HMOs, patients have turned both to legislators and to the courts to prevent the reduction.

- If we try to reduce the intensity of the resources used in providing services, patients, providers, and producers alike will oppose the reductions. Patients view the latest, high-tech treatment as the only acceptable alternative. A clear case in point has been the reaction to limitations on the use of bone marrow transplantation for the treatment of metastatic breast cancer. The treatment is hugely expensive. It is not totally clear that the treatment offers substantial advantages over conventional cancer treatments. Nevertheless patients and their families have obtained tens of millions of dollars in court judgments against insurers who would not approve the treatment. Physicians also frequently oppose constraints on the use of technology in providing service. Producers such as pharmaceutical manufacturers are adamantly opposed to formal limitations on the way physicians use medications.

- There have been numerous attempts to reduce the cost of care by reducing the amount we pay for specific services. Most recently these attempts at cost control have been through limitations in the amount physicians and hospitals are paid for providing care. Both HMOs in the private market for care and government programs such as Medicare and Medicaid have reduced or restricted the amount they are willing to pay health care providers. These reductions have begun to have serious impacts on many of these providers, especially hospitals. A number of large hospitals have faced severe financial difficulties as a result of these payment reductions. In addition a number of physician groups have responded to further reductions in reimbursement by refusing to see patients covered by these insurance plans.

A powerful social force acting against health care reform is the tremendous heterogeneity of American society. Often gains by one segment of society are perceived as a loss by another segment, and thus are resisted. However, as the Figure 12.2 equation illustrates, our need both to expand health care coverage and contain costs will necessitate some form of limitations on the amount of health care we make available. Unfortunately, for those who currently have few limits on the amount of health care available, the imposition of new limits is seen as rationing of care. The very concept of rationing in health care seems somehow to be fundamentally un-American.

Health Care Rationing: Is It Inevitable? Can It Be Acceptable?

In order to understand the concept of health care rationing we again look at the one explicit, federally sanctioned experiment in health care rationing in the United States: the Oregon Health Plan for Medicaid, discussed in Chapter 6. Figure 12.3 again illustrates the fundamental concept behind the plan.

Percent of Poverty Level	Level of Service Available
100	1..50..100..150..200..250..300..350..400..450..500..550..600..650..700
90	1..50..100..150..200..250..300..350..400..450..500..550..600..650..700
80	1..50..100..150..200..250..300..350..400..450..500..550..600..650..700
70	1..50..100..150..200..250..300..350..400..450..500..550..600..650..700
60	1..50..100..150..200..250..300..350..400..450..500..550..600..650..700
50	1..50..100..150..200..250..300..350..400..450..500..550..600..650..700
40	1..50..100..150..200..250..300..350..400..450..500..550..600..650..700
30	1..50..100..150..200..250..300..350..400..450..500..550..600..650..700
20	1..50..100..150..200..250..300..350..400..450..500..550..600..650..700
10	1..50..100..150..200..250..300..350..400..450..500..550..600..650..700

Level of Service Available

Figure 12.3 The Oregon Health Plan for Medicaid: Rationing Care Based on Need

The Oregon state government decided that it was better for low-income people in Oregon and better for the state overall to reallocate some health care funds. By explicitly withholding some services from Medicaid beneficiaries, the funds thus saved were redirected to provide broader (albeit limited) coverage to all those under the poverty line. Health services were rationed so that more could benefit from basic coverage.

What is rationing? Rationing is the prioritized allocation of scarce resources. During World War II, certain foods and industrial raw materials were in scarce supply. There weren't enough of these scarce resources both to supply the war effort and to meet the needs of the civilian population. Under government direction, these scarce resources were allocated on a prioritized basis. The military often had first priority. Those in the civilian pop-

Concept 12.1

Rationing involves the prioritized allocation of scarce resources.

ulation who were most in need came next. (Babies got milk; ambulances got tires.) Finally, those resources still available were allocated on an even basis to those remaining. The system of rationing was widely perceived to be both generally fair and in support of a crucial national goal. As such it received wide support.

When Oregon first proposed rationing health care, a number of sources voiced opposition. Rationing of health care, it was argued, was simply not acceptable. It somehow ran contrary to fundamental American principles to ration something so important.

Based on the definition in Concept 12.1, does the Oregon Health Plan (OHP) involve rationing? Yes, it most certainly does. The OHP involves the prioritized allocation of a scarce resource: health care for the poor. It allocates that resource on the basis of need. Those services that provide the highest benefit are provided to all. Those services that provide the lowest benefit are provided to none. Some people forgo services that have a low level of need so that all people can receive those services with a high level of need.

However, the OHP did not create rationing where rationing did not previously exist. It simply shifted public policy from one form of rationing to another form. Look again at the situation that existed in Oregon before the establishment of the OHP, as illustrated in Figure 12.4.

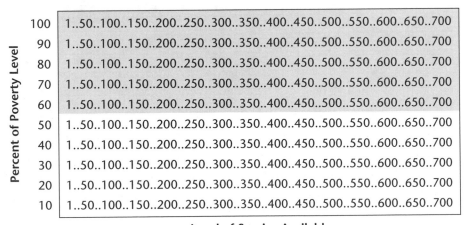

Figure 12.4 Before the Oregon Health Plan for Medicaid: Rationing Care Based on Income

Even before the establishment of the OHP, the Oregon state government approached health care for the poor as a scarce commodity. It prioritized the allocation of Medicaid coverage based on income. Only the very poorest Oregonians—those with incomes below 60% of the poverty line—were covered. In order that the very poorest could receive coverage, those with incomes above this level received no coverage at all.

Before the Oregon Health Plan, Oregon rationed health care to low-income people based on income. After the plan was established, Oregon rationed care based on need. It simply switched from one form of rationing to another. The previous rationing of care was done implicitly, without a formal public decision to do so. The current rationing was done explicitly, after a thorough process of public discussion and debate.

Concept 12.2

The Oregon Health Plan did not create rationing where none previously existed. It instead shifted state policy from rationing health care based on income to rationing care based on need.

The above discussion is about how health care is made available to poor people in Oregon. If instead we look at how health care is made available to people throughout this country, we find the situation illustrated in Figure 12.5.

Percent of Income Level	Level of Service Available
100	1..50..100..150..200..250..300..350..400..450..500..550..600..650..700
90	1..50..100..150..200..250..300..350..400..450..500..550..600..650..700
80	1..50..100..150..200..250..300..350..400..450..500..550..600..650..700
70	1..50..100..150..200..250..300..350..400..450..500..550..600..650..700
60	1..50..100..150..200..250..300..350..400..450..500..550..600..650..700
50	1..50..100..150..200..250..300..350..400..450..500..550..600..650..700
40	1..50..100..150..200..250..300..350..400..450..500..550..600..650..700
30	1..50..100..150..200..250..300..350..400..450..500..550..600..650..700
20	1..50..100..150..200..250..300..350..400..450..500..550..600..650..700
10	1..50..100..150..200..250..300..350..400..450..500..550..600..650..700

Figure 12.5 The Way We Ration Care for the U.S. Population as a Whole

Figure 12.5 illustrates the distribution of health care in the United States in a format similar to the one we used to look at health care in Oregon. The horizontal axis again lists all the services potentially available to people, from the most necessary to the least necessary. (There is of course no actual mechanism to establish such a list for the United States as a whole. For the purposes of discussion we use the ranking of services created for the OHP as if it applied to the entire country.) In this case the vertical axis is not the percentile of the poverty line a person falls into but rather the income percentile at which a person is located. Someone who earned the median income would be at 50%. Low-income people are at low percentiles and high-income people are at high percentiles.

Given the complexity of our insurance system, and the inequity between the very poor who are covered by Medicaid and the somewhat poor who are mostly without health insurance, the diagonal line representing the division between those who are covered and those who are not is not in actuality straight. A truly accurate line would be somewhat zigzagged at the bottom income percentiles. Nonetheless the principle is the same: health care in the United States is distributed largely along income lines. The lower your income, the less care you have available to you. In the United States, as in Oregon before the Oregon Health Plan, we ration health care according to income. We do so, however, implicitly, never having engaged in a public debate about whether we should ration health care and on what basis we should do so.

> ## Concept 12.3
>
> The health care system in the United States involves rationing health care according to income. In contrast to the Oregon Health Plan, this rationing is implicit, with no explicit decision to ration care ever having been agreed to.

In the case of Oregon, why doesn't the state government simply provide enough money to cover all its poor residents with comprehensive health insurance? In the case of the U.S. health care system, why doesn't the federal government adopt a program of full, comprehensive health care, providing all services to all people? The answer in both cases is fairly simple. Oregon simply can't afford to provide all care to all poor people in the state. Similarly, the United States government can't afford to pay for health care for all the people without limitation. Health care has become so expensive that it simply is not feasible for government, whether state or federal, to ensure full access to all services for all people. This inevitable conclusion leads us to Concept 12.4, which states the conundrum of U.S. health care. My students refer to this principle as Barr's law. I offer it with apologies to Abraham Lincoln.

Concept 12.4

You can treat some of the people all of the time (see Figure 12.4), or

You can treat all of the people some of the time (see Figure 12.3), but

You can't treat all of the people all of the time. (Barr's law)

A report in the *New York Times* looked at the problems besetting American health care, and came to a similar conclusion.

> *A major problem with controlling health care costs is that conventional economic principles do not fully apply. Employers want to keep the cost of insurance down to protect their profits. Doctors and hospitals will not perform services at a loss. Drug and insurance companies want the largest profits possible for their shareholders. The less money people pay out of pocket, the more expensive treatments they demand ....*
>
> *So this is the conundrum for politicians. Their constituents will not accept the rationing of their medical treatment. People do not want to be told that good health has a price. On the other hand, neither the politicians nor their constituents want to pay the higher taxes or higher insurance premiums required for unlimited health care. (Rosenbaum 2000)*

To date the United States has been unable to find a solution to this conundrum. Some would say that the problem is not one of being unable, but rather of being unwilling. As a consequence there has been no uniform national policy for access to health insurance. As the cost of providing high-tech, high-quality care has gone up, it has been our national health policy largely to look the other way as more and more people find themselves without health insurance. There have been incremental attempts to address the issue of the uninsured, but we have been unable to agree on a uniform policy approach.

Finding a solution to the three-pointed dilemma of American health care will be extremely difficult. If we are ever to constrain costs, ensure universal access, yet maintain quality, we need to lessen our expectations somewhat about what health care we deserve. As a society we need collectively to agree that in some cases, for some people, we need to forgo certain care that might hold the possibility of some benefit. Recall from our discussion of marginal cost and marginal benefit in Chapter 2 that we often make decisions in health care that we would not make for other types of goods or services. We elect to receive (and have come to expect) many types of care that have a small marginal benefit relative to marginal cost. Since the marginal benefit of that care is small, this implies that forgoing that care would lead to only a small decrement in our health.

Once we as a society come to appreciate health care as a truly scarce commodity, one for which resources are limited, it will become easier for us to accept the form of health care rationing that will be necessary if we are to solve our dilemma. If health care is seen as a zero-sum commodity, it means that any extra care provided to one person will necessarily lead to a reduction in care for someone else. If we are able to accept this conclusion as a principle of our social policy we will be able to develop mechanisms to ensure that we attain a rough level of justice in health care. Our system needs a design, at least for that care financed or regulated publicly, in which no one will be denied care so that someone else may receive care of lesser benefit.

Consistent with our comparison in Chapter 2 of the U.S. and Canadian health care systems, the Canadian system of fully equal access for all is probably not compatible with our national emphasis on the needs of the individual over the needs of the group. Whatever system we adopt will doubtlessly need to allow those with enough money to do so to purchase whatever level of care they wish. If some level of care has small marginal benefit but large marginal cost, but the individual still wants to purchase it with his own money, our system will not be able to prevent that. Rather than adopting the one-class system found in Canada, we will probably need to adopt a form of the two-class system found in Great Britain, where those wishing to buy care outside the National Health Service are free to do so.

Whatever system we adopt will need to incorporate some limits on care, and it will need to be seen as fair. Without widely held perceptions of fairness, few will be willing to forgo care so that someone else may be treated instead. However, recent changes in our American system of care may have made this goal of fairness nearly impossible to attain.

Profit as a Competitor to Cost, Quality, and Access

As discussed in Chapter 7, American health care has undergone a major change over the last 10 to 20 years. Once organized largely on a nonprofit basis, our health care system now includes an increasing number of for-profit corporations: for-profit HMOs, for-profit hospitals, and for-profit medical care providers. This shift to for-profit health care has added a fourth fac-

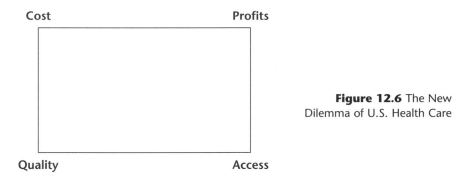

Figure 12.6 The New Dilemma of U.S. Health Care

tor to our national health care dilemma: the need to maintain shareholder profits. This new American health care dilemma is illustrated in Figure 12.6.

Once represented by the three-cornered triangle of cost, quality, and access, the system is now stretched between four points: cost, quality, access, and profit. At nearly every level the issue of profit plays some role in deciding who will get what care. For-profit hospitals have to factor in the need to maintain shareholder return in decisions about which patients to admit, what equipment to buy, and how to measure quality. For-profit insurers must factor shareholder profit into their decisions about how much of the premiums they receive from employers are available for capitation payments to physicians and other providers, and about what types of services and medications will be included under the coverage they offer.

The need to factor profit into decisions about allocating health care dollars is not the only problem with a four-cornered system. As difficult as it may be to somehow find a new equilibrium between cost, quality, and access, the added presence of the profit motive makes finding a comprehensive solution to the problems of U.S. health care nearly impossible.

To understand why this is, consider the patient who has to forgo care so that someone else can receive care of greater marginal benefit. If we are able to create a system of care in which the medical needs of all patients are fairly balanced, patients can have some assurance that their giving up certain care will benefit someone else directly. It may be possible to move to this type of system so long as this assurance can be maintained. In the new, four-cornered American system of care, this assurance cannot be maintained. In a system in which profit competes with quality and access for scarce health care dollars, it is impossible to be certain that money saved by forgoing care of small marginal benefit but large marginal cost will go to providing care to other patients. It may well be the case that money saved in this way provides added profit to shareholders. It is simply not reasonable to expect any patient at any level of income to willingly forgo care, regardless of the cost/benefit profile of that care, if the money saved by doing so will end up going to corporate profit.

I once had as a patient a professor of economics. That professor was upset because his for-profit health insurance company had established a medication formulary, with payment available only for those specific drugs on the list. A medication the professor had previously taken was excluded from the list, and in its place was another, less expensive medication that was equally effective in treating the professor's problem. However, the second medication had some unpleasant (but not dangerous) side effects. I suggested to the professor that a rational economic argument could be made to have only the less expensive medication covered. The marginal benefit of the more expensive drug (fewer side effects) did not justify its substantial marginal cost over the less expensive yet equally effective alternative. The professor, however, contended that issues of marginal cost and marginal benefit were not appropriate when it was his health that was involved. The insurance company had no right, he contended, to withhold the more expensive drug simply to make a profit.

There was little I could offer in response. Were I in his situation, I would probably feel the same way. The presence of the profit motive throughout our health care system makes it unreasonable to expect either individual patients or society as a whole to be willing to move toward an accommodation of the competing needs of cost, quality, and access. So long as we have a system that includes a major role for for-profit corporations, we are unlikely to find a national health policy that can guarantee access to basic, high-quality health care to all people at a cost our society can afford.

Physician Heal Thyself: Physicians and the Profit Motive

Physicians, both individually and collectively, are not strangers to the profit motive. A review of the history of medical practice throughout much of the twentieth century (Starr 1982) reveals that medical practice in this country was historically based on the profit motive: profit for the individual physician. Individual physicians practicing medicine under the fee-for-service system of payment were acting as for-profit entrepreneurs. A physician was not only allowed but encouraged to do everything he could for the patient, so long as he did not harm the patient directly. The more the physician did, the more the physician was paid. For decades there were essentially no limits on how much income a physician could earn, and no one was looking over the physician's shoulder to ask how necessary or appropriate the care was. At that time, however, the incentive to make more profit by providing more care coincided closely with the patient's desire to receive all possible care.

As it turns out, the appropriateness of much of the care provided in the fee-for-service system was questionable. It appears that in many instances physicians were offering if not actually encouraging unnecessary tests and procedures in order to increase their incomes. This history of mixing the economic self-interest of the physician with the medical needs of the patient led George Lundberg, at that time editor of the *Journal of the American Medical Association*, to offer the following warning: "*Caveat aeger*—Let the patient beware" (Lundberg 1995). Dr. Lundberg suggests that few physicians are in medicine just for the money (those he labels "money grubbers") and few exhibit pure altruism (those he labels "altruistic missionaries"). Most physicians are somewhere in between, including at least some level of economic self-interest in their medical decisions. Each physician strikes his or her own balance between the needs of the patient and economic self-interest.

Lundberg suggests that physicians are approximately evenly distributed across a wide spectrum in the way they balance these competing needs. According to his model, this distribution of physicians approximates the shape of the bell-shaped curve, which statisticians refer to as the "standard normal distribution." This curve is illustrated in Figure 12.7.

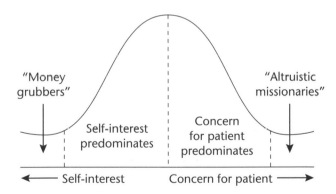

Figure 12.7 The Distribution of Physicians in the United States Along a Scale of Self-Interest Versus Concern for the Patient

Students of statistics will recall that the standard normal distribution has certain characteristics. The mean, median, and mode of the curve are all the same. Ninety-five percent of all points on the curve lie within two standard deviations of the mean.

If Dr. Lundberg's model is correct (and I suspect it is), this would suggest that the medical profession is about equally divided between those situated to the left of the median and those situated to the right of the median. This would mean that, although most physicians attain some type of balance between their own economic needs and the needs of the patient, half of all physicians are more self-interested than they are interested in the benefit of their patients. Few physicians are in it just for the money (those in the left-hand tail of the curve), but likewise few physicians are purely altruistic in their approach to care (those in the right-hand tail of the curve). All the rest of us are situated somewhere between the missionaries and the money grubbers.

This conclusion presents an ethical dilemma for physicians. What steps should we take to ensure that neither physicians' self-interest nor the financial interests of for-profit corporations take precedence over the genuine medical need of patients? In discussing this dilemma Leon Eisenberg suggests that medicine as a profession needs to strengthen and reinforce the culture of professionalism, and in doing so strengthen the commitment of physicians to the needs of their patients. He addresses those of us in the role of teachers and mentors in suggesting,

> It can only promote cynicism among our students if we preach humanism and ignore the realities of the contemporary scene. ... The words "physician" and "patient" are embedded in a proud ethical tradition. Have we always lived up to the ideal we profess? It is obvious that the answer is no. ... No physician could proclaim that the business of medicine is business without losing the respect of her peers. Physicians ought to be advocates for their patients. The best always have been. (Eisenberg 1995)

I suggest that it is up to America's health care professionals, including physicians, nurses, public health analysts, and others, to lead the way toward a system and an ethic that addresses this issue of economic interests and the needs of the patient. Our professional practice should embrace simultaneously the tremendous advances medicine has made in the last 50 years and a genuine commitment to justice in the allocation of health care resources. Part of this concept of justice in health care must be a clear commitment that the needs of the patient come before the financial needs of either individual physicians or health care corporations.

Many of you who are reading this book will be facing these issues and these challenges a very few years from now. The problems addressed by this book will no doubt still exist when you enter your professional careers. I suggest that each of you planning to work either as a physician or in some other capacity in the health care system fully consider the issues raised here. Many factors in society are pushing individual professionals toward the left side of the diagram in Figure 12.7. These forces include the high cost of a professional education, the need to put children through college, or simply the desire to live comfortably. The forces strengthening the right side of the diagram are the ethical tradition of medicine and a commitment to service on behalf of the patient. Every health care professional needs to be aware of this choice.

I propose that each of you choosing to enter the health professions should, from time to time throughout your career, ask the following three questions.

1. Where on this diagram do I want to be situated?

2. In my current professional work, where am I actually situated?

3. Am I willing to do what is necessary to move from where I am now to where I want to be?

REFERENCES

Eisenberg L. Medicine—Molecular, Monetary, or More Than Both? *JAMA* 1995; 274: 331-34.

Fuchs VR. Cost Containment: No Pain, No Gain, and the "Competition Revolution" of the 1980s, pp. 157–86 in Fuchs VR. *The Future of Health Policy*. Cambridge, Mass.: Harvard University Press, 1993.

Lundberg GD. The Failure of Organized Health System Reform—Now What? (*Caveat Aeger*—Let the Patient Beware). *JAMA* 1995; 273:1539–41.

Rosenbaum DE. Swallow Hard; What If There Is No Cure for Health Care's Ills? *New York Times*; September 10, 2000, Section 4, p. 1.

Starr P. *The Social Transformation of American Medicine*. New York: Basic Books, 1982.

residency training
  described, 53–54
  impact of Medicare payment
    formula on, 56–57,
    104–105
Reuther, Walter, 80
"risk adjust" capitation
  premiums (Medicare
  HMOs), 163–164
"risk contracts," 118
RNs (registered nurses), 46
Roosevelt, Franklin, 90
Royal Commission on Health
  Services (1964), 21
RVUs (relative value units),
  100–101

St. Christopher's (hospice), 180
secondary care
  described, 47
  hospitals and, 60–64
  by specialist physicians,
    53–56
Section 1115 Waiver (Social
  Security Act), 118
service plans, 74–76
skilled nursing care, 173–174
social change conditions,
  128–129
Social Security Act (Section
  115), 118
society health, 9–14
specialty physicians
  number of, 51f
  residency training of, 53–54
  rising number of, 54–56
  secondary care by, 53–56
State Children's Health
  Insurance Program (CHIP),
  200–203

statistical bias, 213–214

Tennessee Medicaid managed
  care (Tenncare), 121–1222
tertiary care, 47, 64–65
Thornburgh, Richard, 190–191
Title XIX (Medicaid), 108
Title XVIII (Medicare), 91
Title XXI (CHIP), 200–203
Trudeau, Pierre, 22
Truman, Harry, 90

UCR (usual, customary, and
  reasonable charge), 100
unconscious bias, 214–215
uninsured Americans
  by age (1999), 193f
  characteristics of, 191–195
  CHIP program for children
    of, 200–203
  by household income (1999),
    192f
  low-wage workers/small
    employers as source of,
    195–198, 196f, 197f
  number of, 8–9, 29, 187–189,
    191f
  on-line data sources on, 203
  PPHCA program to reduce
    number of, 198–200
  Wofford vs. Thornburn
    (1991) election focus on,
    190–191
  by work status (1999), 194f
  See also health insurance
United States
  distribution of physicians in,
    235f
  life expectancy in the, 10–11

projected growth in elderly
  population in, 172f
rising cost of health care in,
  5–8, 6t
two perceptions of medical
  profession in, 4t
unique history of health care
  in, 2–4
See also uninsured Americans
U.S. health care system
  comparing Canadian resource
    utilization to, 37t
  cultural institutions driving,
    27–36
  dilemma facing policy makers
    of, 223–225, 224f
  GDP percentage of, 4–5, 7f,
    140f
  high-tech medical treatments
    used in, 32–33
  organizing principles of,
    26–27
  profit dilemma of, 232–234,
    233f
  rationing issue and, 227–232
  rising cost of, 5–8, 6t
  social policy principles of, 27
  unique history of, 2–4
  See also access to care; health
    care
USMGs (United States medical
  schools graduates), 57
utilization review, 142

VA (Veterans' Affairs) health
  system heart study,
  210–212

Wofford, Harris, 190–191, 200